Volume 5 – About Bioethics

FAITH, SCIENCE AND THE ENVIRONMENT

Other titles in the About Bioethics series:

About Bioethics, Volume One: *Philosophical and Theological Approaches* (Connor Court, 2011)

About Bioethics, Volume Two: *Caring for People Who are Sick or Dying* (Connor Court, 2012)

About Bioethics, Volume Three: *Transplantation, Biobanks and the Human Body* (Connor Court, 2012)

About Bioethics, Volume Four: *Motherhood, Embodied Love and Culture* (Connor Court, 2013)

about bi?ethics

FAITH, SCIENCE AND THE ENVIRONMENT

Nicholas Tonti-Filippini

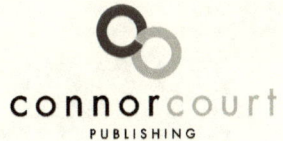

connorcourt
PUBLISHING

Connor Court Publishing Pty Ltd

Copyright © Estate of Nicholas Tonti-Filippini 2017

ALL RIGHTS RESERVED. This book contains material protected under International and Federal Copyright Laws and Treaties. Any unauthorised reprint or use of this material is prohibited. No part of this book may be reproduced or transmitted in any form or by any means, electronic or mechanical, including photocopying, recording, or by any information storage and retrieval system without express written permission from the publisher.

PO Box 7257
Redlands Bay Qld 4165
sales@connorcourt.com
www.connorcourt.com

ISBN: 9781925501513 (pbk.)

Cover design by Ian James

Printed in Australia

Contents

Foreword vii

Acknowledgements x

Preface xi

1. Introduction 1
2. Faith and Creation 9
3. Evolution and the Human Soul 37
   - 3.1 Introduction
   - 3.2 Science and Compatibility with Scripture
   - 3.3 Darwin's Theory
   - 3.4 Genetics and Evolution
   - 3.5 Molecular Biology and Evolution
   - 3.6 Evolution and the Soul
   - 3.7 The Church and Evolution of the Human Soul
   - 3.8 Evolution of the Soul
4. In the Beginning 73
   - 4.1 Creation Out of Nothing
   - 4.2 Doctrine on Creation of the Universe Out of Nothing
   - 4.3 St Thomas Aquinas and Creation
   - 4.4 The Proofs of Creation
   - 4.5 What Does "Creation" Mean?
   - 4.6 Emanation
   - 4.7 The Stability of Creation
   - 4.8 Eternal or Temporal Being
   - 4.9 An Exegesis of Genesis

4.10 Compatibility with Scripture

4.11 Death and the Fall

5. Intrinsic and Instrumental Value and Anthropocentrism 99

5.1 Intrinsic and Instrumental Good

5.2 The Environment and Anthropocentrism

5.3 Dominion and Stewardship

5.4 Is a Creator Logically Necessary?

5.5 The Strength of Our Stewardship

5.6 Teleology

5.7 The Teleology of the Created Order

6. The Goodness of All Creation 123

6.1 The Environment and God's Love

6.2 Christianity and Anthropocentrism

6.3 The Goodness of Creation

7. The Beauty of All Creation 147

7.1 Introduction

7.2 Augustine, Idealism and the Transcendentals

7.3 Matters of Taste

7.4 Other Early Fathers and Beauty

7.5 Aquinas

7.6 The Relationship of Truth, Goodness and Beauty

7.7 Natural Beauty

7.8 Stewardship and Beauty

8. The Sacramentality of Creation: The Invisible in the Visible 176

8.1 Sacraments and Sacramentality

8.2 The Early Fathers and Creation as Witness to the Creator

8.3 Humanity as Witness to God

8.4 Trinitarian Anthropology

8.5 All Creation

8.6 Two Different Ideas of Evolution

8.7 Sin, the Fall and the Sacramentality of All Creation

9. "Brother Wolf": Kinship with Other Species 197

9.1 Introduction

9.2 Peter Singer's Criticisms

9.3 *Imago Dei*

9.4 Evolution, Microbiology and Kinship

9.5 The Saints

9.6 Conclusion

In Memoriam 220

Afterword 222

Appendix A: The Population Question 223

1. Introduction

2. Malthus

3. World Population Rates and Projections

4. Ageing of Developed Populations

5. UN Population Policy

6. The Catholic Church and UN Population Policy

7. Governments and Population Policy

8. Responsible Family Planning

Appendix B: Climate Change 270

Faith, Science and the Environment

1. The Debate in Context
2. The Intergovernmental Panel on Climate Change (IPCC)
3. Human Contribution to Climate Change
4. What Needs to Be Done According to the Experts
5. Criticisms of Climate Change Orthodoxy

Bibliography **288**
Index **303**

Foreword

Sadly, my father passed away before he could see this book published, but we are fortunate that he possessed such an indomitable spirit. Never one to leave a project unfinished, he was still making revisions and updates from the hospital bed where he spent his last month, reading and writing as prolifically and enthusiastically as ever despite the crippling pain and disabilities that eventually claimed his life. The version of this book he left behind on his laptop was essentially complete with the chapters laid out as you see them in the following pages.

In the hour of traumatic stillness following Dad's passing, we, as a family, were confronted with what may be the hardest loss we will ever experience. As I said my silent goodbyes to him in that hospital room, I held his hands for the final time, still as warm and reassuring as ever; so strange to know that his life had just flowed out of them.

I studied them as I sat there beside the bed. Although he was an academic, you wouldn't have known by looking at his hands. They were soft, but also large and scarred, with the thick palms and fingers of a labourer – a fact he was probably proud of. I remember him once talking enviously about the impressive hardened hands of his favourite Volvo mechanic.

Dad's hands had so much life etched into them, so many experiences soaked into the skin. I looked at the gnarled tip of the finger he severed during one of his many constructions in the garage (probably another bookshelf). I could still see the burn marks left by an escaping rope he'd lunged for on that holiday boat trip a few years ago. I thought about the millions of words that passed through those hands, through his pen or onto his keyboard. The hands that had touched so many cricket bats and footballs, the worn handles of hammers and screwdrivers and spanners, the tens of thousands of cups of tea that had been cherished and shared. The hands that had welcomed me and my siblings into the world, no doubt while he wore the huge grin of an elated father. The hands he bragged about once being able to fit around Mum's waist with thumbs and forefingers touching. I won't forget them, those hands, so often framed by the rolled up sleeves of an immaculate business shirt – Dad was a doer and a maker who loved getting his hands dirty, but he always took great pride in his appearance.

In his final years, his hands started to lose feeling and dexterity, and I think that may have upset him the most as his body slowly betrayed him. How he was able to function so well, I'll never be able to understand. He handled the gradual loss of his fitness and ability to walk with so much dignity and resilience. (In fact I think sometimes he secretly enjoyed speeding around on his mobility scooter, and having an excuse to carry around a walking stick.) The increasing debility of his hands seemed to be a much greater frustration, but he still made do, and never once complained about his situation. The pens and keyboards were supplemented with speech recognition software, and the prolific writing continued.

It is odd what your mind clings to in moments of unfathomable grief. For me, a song lyric repeated over and over as I sat there, I couldn't remember where I'd heard it: "These hands are my father's hands, but smaller". I looked at mine next to his, so much smaller and less marked, so callow in comparison. And never was this feeling more apparent to me than when reading this book. The sustained clarity of thought and elegantly constructed arguments he presents in these pages are marvellous to follow. It is an achievement that, when you consider what he suffered during the time of writing, is

Foreword

nothing short of a miracle.

There was another book, a sixth volume, planned for this series based on Dad's lectures regarding Protecting Human Life and Dignity. It was to cover topics such as torture, capital punishment and war. However, the volume was only partially written and I fear, without the presence of Dad's spirit (and hands), we will not see it published.

But in many ways, the book you are holding is a more appropriate end to the About Bioethics series. This volume is a product of Dad's return to his philosophical roots in environmental ethics, as he explores the purpose of the universe and the place of humanity within it.

I won't make any acknowledgements here, as Dad had the humility and presence of mind to make his own before he passed away, but I hope that you will enjoy reading this book as much as I'm sure Dad certainly enjoyed writing it. It is, more than anything, a remarkable testimony to his relentless curiosity and pursuit of the goodness in us all.

Justin Tonti-Filippini

ACKNOWLEDGEMENTS

This is the fifth book in the series and the project has involved many people to whom I am indebted, some of whom have been mentioned in the preface. However, I particularly want to note the contribution made by Bernadette de Bruyn who edited this text. Having disabilities, I have had to rely on dictation software which, though a wonderful assistance on which I am utterly dependent, is far from perfect and having sight difficulties, which make proof reading a skill I no longer possess, meant that there was significant initial editing to be done and Bernadette has done that exactingly and sensitively. I am also grateful to *Vision Australia* for providing the software, a CCTV reader and other assistance, and Dom, Kevin and Ashleigh of the IT department of the Catholic Archdiocese of Melbourne. I thank Dr Anthony Cappello and those who assist him at Connor Court, including the general editor, Michael Gilchrist, for their patience and tolerance. I am also grateful to the students at the John Paul II Institute who first encountered these chapters as lectures and whose feedback helped refine my thinking, and to the faculty at the institute for their encouragement, their scholarly commentary over many lunchtimes, and their willingness to be an audience for student debates and occasionally to make up the even numbers. Finally, I thank Mary and our children whose love sustains me, literally, for without them I would long ago have declared that it was time to surrender to illness and made the decision not to continue with the difficult treatments that sustain my life, including haemodialysis.

Preface

I am very grateful to my students and my colleagues at the John Paul II Institute for sharing the journey with me as I struggled to understand a theology of the environment to match the recent developments in the theology of the body and Trinitarian anthropology. This was a return to a beginning because the first graduate subject that I ever taught was called *Philosophical Approaches to Ecology* within the Graduate School of Environmental Science at Monash University in 1981 and 1982. I am very grateful to the late Professor Hector Munro who proposed that I take over his teaching of the subject and to the late Dr Frank Fisher who died recently. Frank not only made me very welcome in the School but, because he and I shared coping with chronic illness, also greatly encouraged me by his positive attitudes. In particular, his personal commitment to active involvement in the community despite his debilitating illness, which caused him great suffering and inconvenience, and his willingness to mentor me, beyond his teaching and research roles, led me to treat this area as so much more than just an additional teaching task. Frank's commitment to a sustainable environment led him to ride a bike from home, which was to the north of the city of Melbourne, down to Monash University where he worked (a long daily return journey). His illness required him to make frequent use of public toilets along the way and I recall his frustration in finding that the facilities were not maintained or were locked when he needed them. There are many aspects to a sustainable environment!

I recollect teaching classes during the national conflict over the Tasmanian government's decision to build a dam on the Gordon River below the Franklin River (the Franklin Dam). My classes consisted of graduates who were working for industry and thus economically committed to development, not necessarily sustainably, and another group who as passionate environmentalists were often travelling to Tasmania to be part of the protests aimed at stopping the building of the dam. Some years later, I visited the Franklin River valley, with Mary and our young children, and could not help but be relieved that the beautiful Gordon (below Franklin) River was spared, especially when we discovered that Sarah Island was named after Mary's ancestor, Sarah Birch (née Guest). On that trip, all of us were deeply shocked by the effects of open cut mining on the areas around Queenstown and the creation of what looked like a moonscape from what had been forest. At that time I came to understand something of the emotional nature of the debate which for me, up until that time, had been largely academic.

An aspect of this, that a Christian perspective brings, is to seek to view the issues from a perspective of stewardship rather than of self-interest, domination or exploitation. Seeing everything as the fruit of God's creation, and thus the goodness of all creation, is very challenging. When we cut down a tree or cause an animal to be killed for our consumption, or despoil natural beauty for the purposes of construction, there are questions to be answered about the necessity of so doing and the contribution that we are making. This does not mean that we are not justified in making use of the gifts that God has given us. The questions are much more about what constitutes responsible use of the environment and the long-term consequences of the decisions that we implement.

When we had solar panels installed at home and replaced the family car with a pre-loved hybrid, we hoped that in a small way we were shouldering some of the burden of reducing our non-sustainable fuel usage and greenhouse gas emissions and achieving sustainability. However, as it has turned out, neither of these decisions has involved great expense and, in fact, both decisions were financially advantageous at that time and did not involve sacrifice on our part: the car saved a great deal of money on its fuel usage and the return on the solar panels more than paid for them. The much harder decisions to make would involve significant changes in lifestyle to reduce the extraordinary level of consumption expended by our Western lifestyles.

The efforts of our children in volunteering to work and live in developing countries and remote areas have shown us how very much more we need to do before there can be anything like justice in the distribution and use of resources. In the developed world, people like us need to reduce our impact on the environment to sustainable levels.

I am very grateful to Dr Mary Walsh for her love and for the family we have been given and for all that my children, Claire, Lucianne, Justin and John have taught me in these 29 years of parenthood. My students may challenge me with some measure of respect and deference but my children just challenged me. Especially they demanded consistency and had a strong nose for hypocrisy; for that I am deeply grateful and I apologise for all the many ways in which I failed as a parent.

When Mary and I found ourselves alone in the house for a significant time, the first time in 27 years, we felt as though we had just returned after a long survival course. For all that time the dominant reasons for our existence were related to the needs of the children. It is just the way things work for parents. There is both a sense of achievement and a sense of sadness that our task as parents is largely over as the pendulum swings and we ourselves begin to move into a phase of being more the receivers of assistance. The role of being parents was such a rich opportunity. On the other hand, we can now rediscover each other and take up where we left off when that first child arrived and so took over our lives. We look forward to watching our children embark on life's great experiment, being a parent.

One of the joys of being parents is in sharing in the work of creation and realising at first-hand what it is to love and, through love, to be fruitful. Each child, in his or her own way, inherits part of who we are and stands in that extraordinary relationship to us of being the fruit of our love, the embodiment of our love for each other and thus the extension of our gift of love to each other. If we did not appreciate our children, whatever their faults, we would somehow resent ourselves. This lack of appreciation would call into question our participation in the divine work of procreation and, instead, emphasise that we are so flawed by human imperfection, sin and the Fall. The unconditional and unilateral nature of that parental connection seems to reveal the bond that must exist between the Creator of the universe and all creation. Each element of that creation, however small and insignificant or large and grotesque, carries the spark of the Creator's divinity. Each is the subject of divine love.

Appreciating the incredibly delicate and vulnerable nature of ecosystems and the place of each species within them is, in large part, a consequence of science. The scientific story of the Big Bang and the development of the cosmos until finally life forms appeared makes one appreciate the smallness of human history. It is only very late in the history of the cosmos that life forms came to be and the phenomena of mutation and natural selection could, according to the scientific account, begin to do their work of increasing the diversity and functionality of those life forms until sentient beings made their first appearance. Human beings belong to such a very short period, thought to be just 5-6 million years, in the 14 billon year history of the cosmos.

Preface

The scientific account unites us to all creation but it is faith that tells us that all creation is good. As Christians we think of the human person as the pinnacle of that creation, confident that in the significance of the Incarnation is the worthiness of humanity. But some, such as Fr Pierre Teilhard de Chardin, thought that we were still evolving towards Jesus and thus had a way to go to be truly like him. Was Teilhard de Chardin right? Are we still evolving? Others think not, at least in relation to our immortal souls. Popes John Paul II and Benedict XVI accepted the possibility that our bodies probably evolved but they insisted that our immortal souls were instantly and individually created by God. That raises some fascinating challenges for the compatibility of evolutionary theory and creation. There are other challenges also for compatibility. If original sin and death are consequences of the Fall then death did not exist before the Fall. If there were no deaths how did the process of natural selection work? Natural selection works on the basis of change, leading to advantage in the survival and reproduction stakes, and for that to happen there must be selective death.

In this set of essays, I hope to have explained the complexity of the questions that confront us and intend that the discussion should invite readers on a journey of discovery, raising issues that they may not yet have resolved in their own minds or challenging ideas that they thought were settled.

I found this to be a delightful topic precisely because there are so few doctrinal answers and so much theological work to be done. I hope that you share my excitement and joy in exploring the Christian faith and the challenge to theological beliefs that contemporary atheists contend in their claim that science has made God unnecessary.

This task also proved to be an opportunity to explore some of the work of the Early Fathers, the medieval mystics and the medieval rationalists. How does one interpret Augustine in the light of contemporary science? In relation to cruelty to animals, which of the differing views of St. Thomas Aquinas and St Francis of Assisi is to be preferred? How did Cardinal John Henry Newman react to the work of his contemporary, Charles Darwin? How did Darwin, who apparently believed in creation of the universe by God, differ from contemporary Darwinists, such as Richard Dawkins and the late Christopher Hitchens, who used Darwin's theory to argue the case for the redundancy of belief in a creator? Does acceptance of Darwin's theory including the refinements of contemporary science, such as genetic science and cosmology (that were virtually unknown to Darwin), imply scientific atheism's acceptance of chance? Must we follow the leadership of Christian fundamentalists who assert gaps in the science and thus the need for intelligent design as an alternative?

If the human body evolved, how do we explain Scriptural beliefs that bodily death is a result of sin and the Fall? If the human body evolved but the human soul did not (as taught by Pope Benedict XVI and Pope John Paul II), how are we to understand the doctrine, which was proclaimed at Vienne, that the human soul forms and informs the matter to become the unity of body and soul that is the human person?

I believe that faith and science are compatible; particularly I value science for what it can tell us about all of creation, including the incredible mystery of human beings. I need no gaps in the scientific account to sustain my faith. Nevertheless there is the very large fact that science cannot tell us: why we exist, our purpose in being. However, examining what science can tell us about all creation reveals something of the nature of the Creator and divine love, even though that understanding is so affected by sin. The account in the Old Testament of God's relationship to humankind offers an explanation of why we each exist and that account is fulfilled in the story of the Incarnation in the New Testament. Jesus's teachings, life, suffering, death and resurrection, the actions of his apostles and the tradition, built by two thousand years of faithful participation in the life of Christ, answer the "why question"; an answer built on faith, hope and love. Faith and reason are a partnership in which each complements the other as we seek to give expression to the love taught to us by Christ, by his word and deed. It is the excitement of exploring that partnership, in the light of the Gospels, that made writing this book such an enjoyable task.

I hope that as a reader you enjoy this travelogue through the issues that so captured me and my students. I thank the latter for their contributions to my thinking through classroom discussion and the formal graduate student debates that so entertained faculty and friends.

> In the beginning was the Word, and the Word was with God, and the Word was God. He was in the beginning with God; all things were made through him, and without him was not anything made that was made. In him was life, and the life was the light of men. The light shines in the darkness, and the darkness has not overcome it.[1]
>
> ... The Word became flesh and made his dwelling among us. We have seen his glory, the glory of the one and only Son, who came from the Father, full of grace and truth.[2]

---

1 John 1:1-5
2 John 1:14

1
INTRODUCTION

This book explores the relationship between humanity and the environment in the light of contemporary science and a Christian understanding of creation and redemption. Compatibility between Darwin's theory of evolution and the Christian doctrine of creation is discussed. This includes the challenge set us by both Benedict XVI and John Paul II in having accepted the probability of the scientific account of the evolution of the human body but not accepting that the human immortal soul evolved.

The contemporary issues of climate change, population growth, human damage to the environment and the relationship between faith and science are explored by applying the ideas of the goodness, beauty and sacramentality of all creation and other ideas within the Christian tradition, focussing particularly on the contributions of the Early Fathers, such as Augustine and John Chrysostom, and the medieval thinkers, including Albert the Great, Thomas Aquinas and Francis of Assisi, and taking into account the effects of Hellenism on both the Jewish and Christian traditions.

The significance of the belief that the universe is created by God is considered in the context of contemporary scientific theories about the origins of the universe, the nature of the universe and the human place within it. Of particular moment is whether the environment and non-human beings are valued intrinsically or merely instrumentally and whether, historically, Christianity is guilty as charged for fostering an anthropocentric view of the universe, and hence an instrumental view of the environment and of other creatures. This allegation is discussed in the context of faith; seeing all creation, including our scientific understanding of nature, as a witness to the divine Creator, a God who loves us so much that he respects our free will and appoints us stewards of all creation.

This text arose from a series of lectures for a new graduate subject, "Ethics, Creation and the Environment". The subject proved to be popular with students and they participated enthusiastically in a debate on the topic: *"The scientific theory of evolution is the most plausible account of the origins of man and is compatible with the biblical notion of creation and the idea that we are each individually created by God."*

The tension between the biblical account of creation in the book of Genesis and the scientific account of a universe that began 14 billion years ago is not in fact new. In the fifth century, St Augustine had addressed the issue of the impracticality of a too literal reading of Genesis. Nevertheless, there are challenges, in the scientific account of the evolution of the human and animal species, to our understanding of the nature of the human person, the relationship between soul and body, and what happens at both conception and death.

If death is a result of sin and the Fall, how could there have been natural selection, which depends on death, selective survival and reproduction? If the human person is a unity of body and soul, in which the soul forms and informs the matter that is the person, how could the human body have resulted from evolution? These questions are the topic of Chapters 2, 3 and 4, and the answers offered may surprise you, given that the author believes in both Scripture and the probability of the scientific account of the origins of the universe and of humanity.

The contemporary debate over climate change has been divisive in our community. In one sense, the debate has been extraordinarily disappointing because the objectivity of science seems to have been sacrificed to political ideology. The Intergovernmental Panel on Climate Change (IPCC) proved to be disappointing to the extent that, instead of simply reviewing the evidence and presenting us scientific findings, the panel entered into lobbying for a particular political conclusion. As a result, without a politically impartial arbiter of the competing scientific claims, it has been difficult for the ordinary person to interpret the claims made about the occurrence of global warming and the extent to which any rise in temperature is due to a human contribution through carbon emissions into the atmosphere. At the same time, most would recognize, as a general principle, that we should not leave the planet in a worse state for future generations than we received it. Pollution of the environment and the non-sustainable use of materials, such as fossil fuels, are obvious ways in which we do harm to the natural heritage of future generations.

There has also been an economic subtext to the debate. If one accepts that there is a human contribution exacerbating what may be a natural rise in temperature or even only that we need to reduce our non-sustainable use of fossil fuels and pollution of the environment, then, what is the obligation of the present generation to bear the economic cost of adjusting our industries, energy use and way of life in order to lower our levels of carbon emissions, reduce our use of fossil fuels for energy to a sustainable level or eliminate pollution and other forms of degradation of the environment?

Most governments seem to have accepted the science of climate change, that there is a human contribution involved and that climate change is harmful. Also, most accept that we have a responsibility not to pollute the environment and to ensure that our energy use is sustainable. However, the setting of moderate targets in these respects may imply an acceptance that future generations will carry a greater burden of economic cost for environmental damage than this generation. There are also questions about whether carbon trading will simply lead to the developed world paying the developing world to make the sacrifices, especially to life style, that we seem unwilling to make.

Recently, the discussion of climate change and carbon emissions has, to a significant extent, dominated discussion of environmental issues. The issue of sustainable use of energy and other resources, especially the finite nature of fossil fuel reserves, seems to have faded in significance, as have issues such as forest and habitat preservation, loss of species, the effects of inadequately planned land use and pollution generally of land, water and the atmosphere. Whatever happened to the concerns so well explained by Rachel Carson in *Silent Spring*?[1] For my generation, Carson documented the detrimental effects of pesticides on the environment, particularly on birds. She and others showed us that our choices and lifestyles might not be sustainable and the significance of polluting our environment. Global warming and greenhouse theories were not so dominant.

Whatever may be said of the science of human contribution to climate change, the issues of environmental sustainability, the preservation of other species and our relationship to the rest of creation remain matters that Christians need to address. Looking at the Christian tradition as a whole, there does seem to be a distinct difference between the attitudes of the Early Church Fathers and the Christian attitudes of more recent times in regard to the rest of creation. The Christian attitudes that dominated during the industrial revolution seemed to treat the environment as an unlimited resource. The idea that we might do irreparable damage, or that the level of resource use was unsustainable in the long-

---

1 Rachel Carson, *Silent Spring*, Boston, Goughton Mifflin, 1962.

term, did not seem to be a significant part of Christian thinking other than for those few who, like Malthus, took the view that ultimately there would be a problem of overpopulation. During the industrial revolution there did not seem to be strong support for the opinion that we needed to be concerned about our use of the environment and natural resources.

There are instrumental reasons for preserving species and their habitats, such as the future use of biodiversity, and what is called the "museum argument" which proposes that future generations not be deprived of their opportunities to appreciate the diversity of species and natural wonders, including our wildernesses. On the other hand, appreciation of the sacramentality and beauty of all creation, such as was expressed by the Early Fathers and in the Middle Ages by such as St Francis of Assisi, provides reason for Christians to value all creation for intrinsic reasons and not just instrumentally. There are also issues to do with the extent that human beings can affect evolutionary processes and even make their own changes to plant, animal or human genetic determinants of life forms. We are capable of turning the scientific abilities upon ourselves and altering our progeny. Should the human person be seen as an artefact or an icon?[2] Is the human genome sacred?[3] Should we respect the genetic integrity of animal species?[4]

This book seeks to explore intrinsic and instrumental reasons for treating the rest of creation in the light of stewardship rather than domination and exploitation. In his Peace Day message of

---

[2] Reverend Robert Brungs, 'The Human Body: Artefact or Icon?', *Proceedings of the 1983 Annual Conference of St Vincent's Bioethics Centre*, eds. J.N. Santamaria and N. Tonti-Filippini, Melbourne, 1983.

[3] I have addressed this question in 'Xenotransplantation and Human-Animal Transgenesis', in *About Bioethics Volume III: Transplantation, Biobanks and the Human Body*, Ballan, Connor Court, 2012, pp. 97-118 (also published in the *National Catholic Bioethics Quarterly*, Volume 6, No. 4, Winter 2006).

[4] Pontifical Academy for Life, 'Prospects for Xenotransplantation: Scientific Aspects and Ethical Consideration', *L'Osservatore Romano*, 26 September 2001.

1990, *Peace with God, Peace with All Creation*, Pope John Paul II offered a very challenging approach to recognizing that Christ came to save, not just humanity, but all creation. This implies that our stewardship of the environment is more than just a matter of utility for future generations but that it should be reflective of the sacredness and goodness of all that God has made.

So after exploring, in Chapters 2, 3 and 4, the relationship between faith and science and the debates over evolution and creation, Chapter 5 addresses the matter of the distinction between intrinsic and instrumental value and anthropocentrism. Then Chapter 6 explores the goodness of all creation and Chapter 7 studies the beauty of all creation.

The discussion of these transcendentals, as we experience them in the natural world, leads on to Chapter 8 which considers the extent to which all creation is a witness to the Creator – what is known as the sacramentality of all creation. By studying creation, including ourselves, we can deepen our understanding of the divine Creator who brought us into being and sustains us. What are we to make of modern Christian writers, such as Fr Pierre Teilhard de Chardin, and their ideas that human beings are continuing to evolve towards Christ?

Sharing the planet with us are millions of other species, many of whom demonstrate some level of sentience. How are we to understand their suffering? What is the meaning of our stewardship and dominion over other creatures? In our tradition we have both St Francis and St Thomas Aquinas. Are their views about other animals able to be reconciled? The Australian Broadcasting Corporation televised a current affairs report on Australian cattle being exported to Indonesia for commercial slaughter for consumption purposes. The report's graphic portrayal of cruelty to those animals led to a dramatic decision in 2011 by the Labor Government, led by the Honourable Julia Gillard, to temporarily cease the live export trade to Indonesia. The government seemed to react to the effect of the program on public opinion about the depiction of cruelty to animals. At the time, there did not seem to be obvious Christian leadership on the issue. The Churches seemed to be absent from the debate. Was that because cruelty to animals does not figure very highly in terms of Christian priorities? Was it that we were simply ignored and our opinions not considered worth reporting by the media, or was it that we really did not have anything to say? Were we so concerned about Christian/Islamic relations that we did not want to be seen to say anything that might appear religiously divisive? What views do Christians have about animal cruelty? These matters are discussed in Chapter 9, *"Brother Wolf": Kinship with Other Species?*, including the approach taken to the issue by writers such as Peter Singer of *Animal Liberation* fame.[5]

In Appendix A, *The Population Question*, the issue of a limited environment and an ever expanding population, which has exercised intelligent minds throughout our history, both ancient and modern, is explored once again in the light of contemporary science but with the added analysis of what has happened when governments and others tried to control population growth. The contemporary phenomena of birth rates, substantially below population replacement levels, and the development of gender imbalance indicate the economic and social considerations required, from those who are making and implementing policy, to allow freedom to parents to make informed decisions about their own parenting rather than to be coercive. The evidence suggests that finding solutions to poverty, caused by the maldistribution of resources and the lack of education, would seem to suggest more humane goals and more effective ways of addressing the effects

---

5 Peter Singer, *Animal Liberation: Towards an End to Man's Inhumanity to Animals*, Paladin Books, 1977.

of population growth and threats to the environment than coercive policies in relation to family size.

Appendix B, *Climate Change*, addresses the contemporary problem of human contributions to climate and includes discussion of the dangers posed by the science threatening its own credibility as it seeks to influence policy. The evidence suggests that when government scientists became involved in policy development and the implementation of that policy, the community began to lose confidence in their reportage and modelling. The ordinary lay person became more sceptical about competing scientific claims on the many sides of the debate and for many that scepticism, which is an important part of scientific advancement, became cynicism. Cynicism is not helpful to our community in determining what responsible behaviour on this issue is because cynicism undermines legitimate authority, making all claims equally lacking in credibility.

I hope you enjoy this work which I found to be challenging, enjoyable and enormously informative as I set about trying to understand the tradition well enough to be able to teach it.

2
FAITH AND CREATION

Genesis gives an account of our origin and science has given another. The Genesis story maintains that God created the world and all creation within six days. Science tells of the evolution of species over millennia. Genesis tells us of our relationship to God and how that relationship gives us purpose. Genesis does not tell us how God created us: what is not significant is the chronology. Science on the other hand seeks to explain how we originated but not why we originated. It cannot tell us of God's love for us, that He created us out of love so that we can love Him. It cannot explain who in fact we are - that we are persons made in God's image and likeness. Principally this is what the Genesis story is about.

The approach that the Catholic Church has taken to the science is not to challenge it. Science and religion are not in collision, they are operating in different spheres. The Church learned a grave lesson when it insisted against Galileo in relation to his support of the scientific theory which, based on observation and mathematics, maintained that in fact the earth rotated around the sun.

Finding themselves dispossessed of the land, the holy writers of the first account in Genesis had to reconcile their idea of God with the experience of dispossession. Such was not the account given by the writers of the second account in Genesis; nor is the creation of the world in a week the account of creation implied by the writers of the Psalms. The task of Scripture scholars is to try seek consistency, in order to reconcile the differences, and the whole of Scripture itself is an evolving story that only has its fulfilment, and hence its meaning, in the Incarnation. In Jesus we have the completion of the message that God had been giving us throughout our history.[6]

The crucial aspects of that first account are of a creator who loves us and who brings us into being out of love for us and in order that we might love Him. Holy Scripture is thus an account of the relationship between the Creator and His Creation and of humanity, made in His image and likeness, with the inherent capacity for rationality. The physical realities that are addressed by science are part of an unfolding story also, as science builds upon the fruits of its own project. The early writers of Scripture were no doubt influenced by their knowledge of the physical world and explained God's actions in the light of that knowledge. Unsurprisingly, there is a lack of consistency in their assumptions about the physical world; there is also evolution of their knowledge of the Creator because their understanding needed the Jesus event to complete it.

It would therefore be odd if the Church were to take the understanding of the physical world possessed by the holy writers and demand of it the consistency that one would expect of a well formed and substantiated scientific theory. This would be to demand too much of the holy writers. Theirs was a developing task and one which, in their own time, was very incomplete. What is evident to us is that God uses very ordinary means to communicate His relationship and His love for us. The background to the developing understanding of the physical reality in which they found themselves is not the essential message. It is a background, and just that, for the story of God's love and His loving purpose for His creation.

Faced with the puzzles of these two very different branches of

---

6 Joseph Cardinal Ratzinger, *'In the beginning ...' A Catholic Understanding of the Story of Creation and the Fall*, Eerdmans, 1995.

human thinking, the natural sciences and theology, in 1950, Pope Pius XII wrote cautiously in his encyclical *Humani Generis*:

> The Teaching Authority of the Church does not forbid that, in conformity with the present state of human sciences and sacred theology, research and discussions, on the part of men experienced in both fields, take place with regard to the doctrine of evolution, insofar as it inquires into the origin of the human body as coming from pre-existent and living matter.[7]

On October 23, 1996, after a further 46 years of the gathering of evidence, including immense discoveries such as DNA and the mechanics of cell function, and confirmation of the processes of evolution, Pope John Paul II said in a speech to the Pontifical Academy of Sciences:

> Today, almost half a century after the publication of the encyclical, new knowledge has led to the recognition of the theory of evolution as more than a hypothesis. It is indeed remarkable that this theory has been progressively accepted by researchers, following a series of discoveries in various fields of knowledge. The convergence, neither sought nor fabricated, of the results of work that was conducted independently is in itself a significant argument in favor of this theory.
>
> A theory is a meta-scientific elaboration, which is distinct from, but in harmony with, the results of observation. With the help of such a theory a group of data and independent facts can be related to one another and interpreted in one comprehensive explanation. The theory proves its validity by the measure to which it can be verified. It is constantly being tested against the facts; when it can no

---

[7] Pope Pius XII, *Humani Generis*, 12 August 1950. http://www.newadvent.org/library/docs_pi12hg.htm#36 (accessed 2010-2014).

longer explain these facts, it shows its limits and its lack of usefulness, and it must be revised.[8]

In other words, the Catholic Church had understood that the account of the origins of life in Scripture was varied and developing from the outset and capable of absorbing and adapting to the growth in human knowledge, as it can be expected to do in the future. However this does not challenge what is central to the Scriptural account of all its writers – their understanding of the loving relationship between God and His creation. Thus the Church did not respond to the idea of evolution negatively but supported the efforts of science to explain our origins and, as the science developed greater evidence for the theory, the Church has expressed willingness to be guided by the evidence. This has not been the case for all Christians. The response of the Church of England at the time was mixed, with some theologians supporting the theory and others being critical. The most prominent critic was the Bishop of Oxford, Samuel Wilberforce, who ridiculed the idea that we might be descended from apes. Darwin himself considered it "absurd to doubt that a man might be an ardent theist and an evolutionist".[9] In publishing the *Origin of the Species,* he did not propose that his theory would be a vehicle for atheism.

Clearly if we are to take the Genesis account to be an historical record of our biological origins then there is a conflict in Scripture between science and faith. In relation to this seeming contradiction Pope Benedict XVI explains:

> We cannot say: creation *or* evolution, inasmuch as these two things respond to two different realities. The story of the dust

---

8 Pope John Paul II, *Truth Cannot Contradict Truth,* 22 October 1996. http://www.newadvent.org/library/docs_jp02tc.htm (accessed 9 June 2011).
9 Charles Darwin, letter to J. Fordyce on 7 May 1879, 'Letter no. 12041', *Darwin Correspondence Project,* http://www.darwinproject.ac.uk/entry-12041 (accessed 2010-2014).

of the earth and the breath of God, which we just heard [the Genesis account], does not in fact explain *how* human persons come to be but rather *what they are*. It explains their inmost origin and casts light on the project that they are. And, vice versa, *the theory of evolution seeks to understand and describe biological developments*. But in so doing it cannot explain where the "project" of human persons comes from, nor their inner origin, nor their particular nature. To that extent we are faced here with two complementary – rather than mutually exclusive – realities.[10]

Pope Benedict XVI went on to say:

It is the affair of the natural sciences to explain how the tree of life in particular continues to grow and how new branches shoot out from it. This is not a matter for faith. But we must have the audacity to say that the great projects of the living creation are not the products of chance and error. Nor are they the products of a selective process to which divine predicates can be attributed in illogical, unscientific, and even mythic fashion. *The great projects of the living creation point to a creating Reason and show us a creating Intelligence*, and they do so more luminously and radiantly today than ever before. Thus we can say today with a new certitude and joyousness that the human being is indeed a divine project, which only the creating Intelligence was strong and great and audacious enough to conceive of. *Human beings are not a mistake but something willed; they are the fruit of love*. They can disclose in themselves, in the bold project that they are, the language of the creating Intelligence that speaks to them and that moves them to say: Yes, Father, you have willed me.[11]

---

10 Ratzinger, *'In the beginning ... '*, op. cit.
11 Ibid

This response is quite different from those who pursue the notion of "intelligent design" which has been referred to in the following way:

> Intelligent design refers to a scientific research program as well as a community of scientists, philosophers and other scholars who seek evidence of design in nature. The theory of intelligent design holds that certain features of the universe and of living things are best explained by an intelligent cause, not an undirected process such as natural selection. Through the study and analysis of a system's components, a design theorist is able to determine whether various natural structures are the product of chance, natural law, intelligent design, or some combination thereof. Such research is conducted by observing the types of information produced when intelligent agents act. Scientists then seek to find objects which have those same types of informational properties which we commonly know come from intelligence. Intelligent design has applied these scientific methods to detect design in irreducibly complex biological structures, the complex and specified information content in DNA, the life-sustaining physical architecture of the universe, and the geologically rapid origin of biological diversity in the fossil record during the Cambrian explosion approximately 530 million years ago.[12]

The Catholic Church has no difficulty with the idea that we may have evolved from other species or that the process of evolution may have occurred through mechanisms of natural selection and mutation.

The notion of intelligent design risks being something

---

12 Discovery Institute – Center for Science and Culture, 'What is intelligent design?', *Intelligent Design*, http://www.intelligentdesign.org/whatisid.php (accessed 2010-2014).

of a "God of the Gaps". The term goes back to a 19th century evangelist, Henry Drummond, taken from his Lowell Lectures on the *Ascent of Man*. He is critical of those who point to the things that science cannot yet explain – "gaps which they will fill up with God" – and urges them to embrace all nature as God's, "... an immanent God, which is the God of Evolution, is infinitely grander than the occasional wonderworker, who is the God of an old theology."[13]

This view was taken by other leading Christians such as Dietrich Bonhoeffer, who wrote:

> ... how wrong it is to use God as a stop-gap for the incompleteness of our knowledge. If in fact the frontiers of knowledge are being pushed further and further back (and that is bound to be the case), then God is being pushed back with them, and is therefore continually in retreat. We are to find God in what we know, not in what we don't know.[14]

Just three years after Darwin published the *Origin of the Species*, Cardinal John Henry Newman clearly accepted the possibility of evolutionary theory on similar grounds:

> There is as much want of simplicity in the idea of the creation of distinct species as in that of the creation (of) trees in full growth (whose seed is in themselves), or of rocks with fossils in them. I mean that it is as strange that monkeys should be so like men, with no "historical connection" between them as that there should be the notion that there was no history ... of facts by which fossil bones got into rocks ... I will either go whole hog with

---

[13] Thomas Dixon, *Science and Religion: A Very Short Introduction*, Oxford University Press, 2008, p. 45.
[14] Dietrich Bonhoeffer, letter to Eberhard Bethge on 29 May 1944, *Letters and Papers from Prison*, E. Bethge (ed.) and R.H. Fuller (trans.), Touchstone, 1997, pp. 310-312.

Darwin or, dispensing with time and history altogether, hold, not only the theory of distinct species but that also of the creation of the fossil-bearing rocks.[15]

Later he wrote:

> Men are impatient, and for precipitating things; but the Author of Nature appears deliberate throughout His operations, accomplishing His natural ends by slow successive steps. And there is a plan of things beforehand laid out, which, from the nature of it, requires various systems of means, as well as length of time, in order to the carrying on its several parts into execution. Thus, in the daily course of natural providence, God operates in the very same manner as in the dispensation of Christianity, making one thing subservient to another; this, to somewhat farther; and so on, through a progressive series of means, which extend, both backward and forward, beyond our utmost view. Of this manner of operation, everything we see in the course of nature is as much an instance as any part of the Christian dispensation.[16]

The following letter from Newman explains his acceptance of evolution and how much more we can appreciate a God who created a universe that evolves. He expresses appreciation for a God who works in this way, creating something that would develop rather than is formed from the outset, and draws an analogy between ordinary reproduction of a child from parents and evolution. It is so delightfully succinct I have included it and its important postscript in full:

---

15 John Henry Newman, *The Philosophical Notebook of John Henry Newman*, vol. II, eds. E. Sillem and A. J. Boekrad, Louvain, 1970, p. 158.
16 John Henry Newman, *An Essay on the Development of Catholic Doctrine*, Longman Green & Co., 1878, pp. 55-98. Available from http://www.newmanreader.org/works/development/index.html (accessed 2010-2014).

John Henry Newman to J. Walker of Scarborough
The Oratory Bm May 22/68
[Birmingham, May 22, 1868]

My dear Canon Walker

I got Smith on the Pentateuch at once on your suggestion, and have been much interested in what I have read of it – but have not read enough to get into it as a whole [W. Smith, *The Book of Moses or the Pentateuch in its Authority, Credibility, and Civilization*, London 1868]. Mr Beverly's work too has come, but with no supplemental chapter. Pray convey my acknowledgement to the *unknown* author [*The Darwinian Theory of the Transmutation of Species examined by a Graduate of the University of Cambridge*, London 1868]. It is a careful and severe examination of the theory of Darwin – and it shows, as is most certain he would be able to do, the various points which are to be made good before it can cohere. I do not fear the theory so much as he seems to do – and it seems to me that he is hard upon Darwin sometimes, which [sic] he might have interpreted him kindly. It does not seem to me to follow that creation is denied because the Creator, millions of years ago, gave laws to matter. He first created matter and then he created laws for it – laws which should *construct* it into its present wonderful beauty, and accurate adjustment and harmony of parts *gradually*. We do not deny or circumscribe the Creator, because we hold he has created the self acting originating human mind, which has almost a creative gift; much less then do we deny or circumscribe His power, if we hold that He gave matter such laws as by their blind instrumentality moulded and constructed through innumerable ages the world as we see it. If Mr Darwin in this or that point of his theory comes into collision with revealed truth, that is another matter –

but I do not see that the *principle* of development, or what I have called construction, does. As to the Divine *Design*, is it not an instance of incomprehensibly and infinitely marvellous Wisdom and Design to have given certain laws to matter millions of ages ago, which have surely and precisely worked out, in the long course of those ages, those effects which He from the first proposed. Mr Darwin's theory *need* not then to be atheistical, be it true or not; it may simply be suggesting a larger idea of Divine Prescience and Skill. Perhaps your friend has got a surer clue to guide him than I have, who have never studied the question, and I do not [see] that 'the accidental evolution of organic beings' is inconsistent with divine design – It is accidental to *us*, not to *God*.

Most sincerely yours in Xt John H Newman

P.S. Why is not the principle of generation atheistic, if that of development is? Did we not know the *fact* that species and races are drawn out in succession from one couple, we might say that it was a theory inconsistent with the doctrine of creation. And à fortiori, it might be urged, 'here the *accidental* meeting and marriage of two persons, or the sinful intercourse, will oblige the Almighty to create a soul at any moment.' Therefore (not only not the body, but) the soul is *not* created, but is the accidental consequence of the human will, etc. etc.[17]

This view is adopted by Dr George Coyne SJ, the Director of the Vatican Observatory, who argues:

1. The Intelligent Design movement, while evoking a God of power and might, a designer God, actually belittles God, makes her/him too small and paltry;

---

17 John Henry Newman, letter to J. Walker of Scarborough on May 22 1868, 'The Oratory Bm May 22/68', *The Letters and Diaries of John Henry Newman*, vol. XXIV, eds. C.S. Dessain and T. Gornall, Oxford, Clarendon Press, 1973, pp. 77-78.

2. Our scientific understanding of the universe, untainted by religious considerations, provides for those who believe in God a marvellous opportunity to reflect upon their beliefs.[18]

Coyne suggests that we take the results of modern science seriously and concludes that if we do then we will envisage a God who made a universe that has within it a certain dynamism and thus participates in the very creativity of God. He argues that such a view of creation can be found in early Christian writings, especially in those of St. Augustine in his comments on Genesis.[19] God is more like a parent or one who speaks encouraging and sustaining words. Scripture is very rich in these thoughts. It presents, indeed anthropomorphically, a God who gets angry, who disciplines, who nurtures the universe. Thus theologians already possess the concept of God's continuous creation. The universe has a certain vitality of its own like a child does. It has the ability to respond to words of endearment and encouragement. You discipline a child but you try to preserve and enrich the individual character of the child and her own passion for life. A parent must allow the child to grow into adulthood, to come to make her own choices, to go her own way in life. Words which give life are richer than mere commands or information. In such ways does God deal with the universe.[20]

On this basis Coyne argues that Intelligent Design diminishes God, by making God a designer rather than a lover. Those who advocate Intelligent Design seem to be hoping for the durability of gaps in our scientific knowledge of evolution, so that they

---

18 Reverend George V. Coyne, 'Science Does Not Need God. Or Does It?', lecture presented at the American Enterprise Institute, 21 Oct 2005, http://home.comcast.net/~pdnoerd/DrCoyneTalk.pdf (accessed 2010-2014).
19 St Augustine, *The Literal Meaning of Genesis (De Genesi ad Litteram)*, in J.H. Taylor (trans.), *Ancient Christian Writers* 41-42, New York, Newman Press, 1982.
20 Coyne, op. cit.

can fill them with God. God is thus imported to explain things that we cannot explain otherwise. God is thus seen as a response to that need. But God is not a response to our need. Rather, the God who created an evolving universe, in his infinite freedom, continuously creates a world which reflects freedom at all levels of the evolutionary process to a greater and greater complexity. God lets the world be what it will be in its continuous evolution. He does not intervene but rather allows, participates, loves.[21]

Importantly, Coyne rejects the idea that evolutionary theory means a commitment to chance. Whether some proponents of the theory have described the evolution of life, and human life in particular, as a chance event is not the issue. The theory of evolution is simply the claim that life and the variety of species have evolved, with more complicated life forms having evolved from less complicated life forms and even at some stage from non-living matter. We do not know the precise mechanism of that evolution. Various theories are offered for mutation and Charles Darwin has offered an account of the effects of evolution whereby certain aspects that provide an advantage in particular environments and changing circumstances are selected. The particular organic structures that form what we know as life are thought to have originated through the right molecules meeting in precisely the right circumstances. In fact the story of the cosmos first developing life forms is possibly a more difficult event to understand or explain than the evolution of species.

The empirical data to support evolutionary theory, with respect to biotic evolution, comes from various independent scientific enterprises, including molecular biology, palaeontology and comparative anatomy. Coyne points to the facts that, according to contemporary understanding, the universe is 13.7 billion years old

---

21 Ibid.

and it contains about 100 billion galaxies, each of which contains 100 billion stars of an immense variety. The fact that there are billions of stars, he argues, makes it such that the interplay of chance, necessity and opportunity leads inevitably to life and intelligence.[22]

That is to say God was not playing with chance. He knew that mankind would evolve from this process. Similarly, Albert Einstein once said, "It seems hard to sneak a look at God's cards. But that He plays dice and uses 'telepathic' methods ... is something that I cannot believe for a single moment."[23]

Stephen Hawking disagrees:

> God is bound by the Uncertainty Principle, and cannot know both the position, and the speed, of a particle. So God does play dice with the universe. All the evidence points to him being an inveterate gambler, who throws the dice on every possible occasion.[24]

Quoting from St Basil, Pope Benedict XVI suggests that some people, "deceived by the atheism they bore within them, imagined that the universe lacked guidance and order, at the mercy as it were of chance". The Pope goes on to say:

> How many these "some people" are today! Deceived by atheism they consider and seek to prove that it is scientific to think that all things lack guidance and order as though they were at the mercy of chance. The Lord through Sacred Scripture reawakens our reason which has fallen asleep and tells us: in the beginning was the creative Word. In the beginning the creative Word – this Word that created

---

22 Ibid.
23 Albert Einstein in a letter to Cornel Lanczos on 21 Mar 1942, in *Albert Einstein, the Human Side*, eds. B. Hoffman and H. Dukas, New Jersey, Princeton, 1979.
24 Stephen Hawking, 'Does God play Dice?', lecture available at http://www.hawking.org.uk/does-god-play-dice.html (accessed 2010-2014).

all things, that created this intelligent design which is the cosmos – is also love.[25]

The fact that this is an evolving universe, and that we are part of that evolutionary story, is consistent with God having created it with the capacity for unfolding development as part of the design. Even though this happened through natural processes and foreseeable contingencies makes it no less an intelligent design. The claim that Hawking made in relation to the uncertainty principle is based on the scientific theory that there are genuine random events: he refers to particle theory and the difficulty of measuring both the location and speed of a particle at the same time.[26]

I am not a physicist. My father was and understood these things better than me, but I cannot follow the logic that holds that because there are seemingly random events, such as seems to be the case with black holes, therefore not all natural phenomena events can be determined by rules of nature. The argument, it seems to me, makes an inference from observed unpredictability to arbitrary randomness. However, unpredictability would seem to indicate a lack of an explanation or theory rather than that there can be no such explanation. Of course, if Hawking is right, then it would be surprising if there were any contemporary physicists who believed in the possibilities of a created natural order and hence a creator. But there are. Eugene Wigner, a Nobel Prize winner in physics, explained the limitations of contemporary physics and the way in which a theory may be validated by its consistent application to a very small data range, given the extreme relative ignorance of the universe amongst physicists. To make the point he discussed the facts of two theories that conflict, the theory of relativity is

---

25 Pope Benedict XVI, General Audience, 9 Nov 2005, http://www.vatican.va/holy_father/benedict_xvi/audiences/2005/documents/hf_ben-xvi_aud_20051109_en.html (accessed 2010-2014).
26 Hawking, op. cit.

true for macroscopic objects and quantum mechanics is true for microscopic particles, but neither is universally true. He challenged the capacity of contemporary physics to explain materialism.[27] Sir Rudolf Peierls, also a 20th century physicist, said, "... the premise that you can describe in terms of physics the whole function of a human being ... including [his] knowledge, and [his] consciousness, is untenable. There is still something missing."[28]

The existence of order in the cosmos indicates a God who knew that development in its origin, whatever the origin was in His decision to create it, and who has allowed those processes the freedom to develop. God is not like a watchmaker designing and making a final product. Rather the empirical evidence suggests the universe, from the outset, had the capacity to develop immense complexity through its own processes until it could produce us, made in His image and likeness. This image of God as lover rather than designer is a very rich one. God created all that is, all the goodness of the universe, knowing its capacity to evolve and the complexity that would develop within it. The wisdom and the design were in that first act of creation. As Newman expressed it, evolutionary theory suggests "a larger idea of Divine Prescience and Skill".[29]

In summary, Darwin's observations in what is known as his *Theory of Evolution by Natural Selection* are relatively minimal compared to the many claims that are attributed to it, including claims that it supports atheism. The central claims of his theory are:

---

27 Eugene Wigner, 'The Unreasonable Effectiveness of Mathematics in the Natural Sciences', in *Communications in Pure and Applied Mathematics*, vol. 13, No. I (February 1960), New York, John Wiley & Sons, 1960.
28 Sir Rudolf Peierls, interviewed by Paul Davies, transcript in *The Ghost in the Atom*, eds. P.C.W. Davies and J.R. Brown, Cambridge, Cambridge University Press, 1986, p. 75.
29 Newman, *The Letters*, op. cit.

1. Most animals have such high fertility rates that their population size would increase exponentially if all individuals were to reproduce.
2. Yet, except for seasonal fluctuations, populations remain relatively stable in size.
3. Because environmental resources are limited, individuals compete for resources, limiting survival and reproduction.
4. Individual characteristics vary within populations and those members of a population that are better adapted for survival in the face of competition are more likely to pass their characteristics on to the next generation.
5. Thus, species gradually accumulate inherited adaptations that best suit them for their environment, passing these on to progeny. Speciation involves gradually accumulated differentiation of characteristics.[30]

Thus for Darwin, the process of natural selection was the main mechanism of evolution. However natural selection does not explain biodiversity in itself. For that a theory of mutation is required.

Genetic mutation is a common occurrence. Genetic change happens frequently within the one individual, with opportunities for it with each cell replication. There are literally trillions of cells within us, with the average human cell replicating between 40 and 90 times before built-in obsolescence halts the process. Each replication is an opportunity for genetic mutation. There are many factors that can produce changes to the genetic code during replication including those factors known to cause cancer, such as radiation and chemicals in the environment.

---

30 Evolutionist, 'Beyond Darwin and Neo-Darwinism', *Mechanisms of Evolution*, 31 December 2007, http://mechanismsevo.blogspot.com.au/2007/12/beyond-darwin-and-neo-darwinism.html (accessed 2010-2014). (cf. Ernst Mayr, *What Evolution Is*, Basic Books, 2001, p. 116).

We are very familiar with mutation. For instance, cancer involves a mutation of the cells that interfere with the controls over cell replication. Identical twins (monozygotic twins) have difference genetic fingerprints even though they would have begun from the same cell and inherited the same genetic code from their parents. Cell replication is not perfect as it is affected by environmental factors which lead to identifiable genetic or epigenetic changes between identical twins. Many genetic disorders, such as the trisomy disorders (e.g. Downs or Edwards Syndrome), involve a mutation that makes the child genetically different from his or her parents because he or she has an extra chromosome in each cell. In trisomy, during the process of the egg cell being produced, it is thought that, instead of the chromosome being replicated and the cell dividing to form two cells – each with half the range of chromosomes, during the division one cell receives an extra chromosome and the other cell lacks the same chromosome. The latter results in a condition called monosomy (such as Turner Syndrome).

Mutation can also happen through genetic recombination.[31] Eggs and sperm are produced by a process called meiosis in which a new cell is formed which has only half the normal number of chromosomes. During the process chromosomes are paired and a crossover can occur with one part of a chromosome swapping with part of another chromosome and becoming attached to the wrong chromosome.

Genetic mutation can also occur in the replication of ordinary cells in which genetic sequences are "translocated" somewhere else on the chromosome. A gene sequence may also be altered by: "deletion" in which elements may go missing, "insertion" in which

---

31 Rasmus Grønfeldt Winther, 'Systemic Darwinism', *Proceedings of the National Academy of Sciences U.S.A.*, vol. 105 no. 33, 2008, pp. 11833–11838.

an element is added, "inversion" in which an order is "reversed" and "substitution" in which a sequence is replaced by another.[32]

As it is understood, the process of evolution beginning from matter includes:

- the formation of molecules
- the formation of replicating molecules
- compartmentalization, independent replicators
- molecular chains and molecules – chromosomes
- RNA as the first form of genes and enzymes and the formation of a genetic code or ribosome
- DNA and proteins
- Prokaryotes (a single cell organism)
- Eukaryotes (multiple cell organisms)
- asexual reproduction developing to sexual reproduction
- Protists – cell differentiation and developments leading to the formation of fungi, plants and then animals
- individuals living as pairs to form colonies
- primate societies then the development of human societies capable of language, writing, culture ...[33]

Despite our familiarity with mutation and our understanding of the effects of natural selection, Fr Coyne, as a supporter of evolutionary theory, confirms we certainly do not have the scientific knowledge in detail to say how each living creature came to be. We do not know precisely how each more complex chemical system came to contribute to the process of self-organization which brought about the diversity of life forms as we know them today.

---

32 'Genetic Mutations', *Biology Online*, 2000, http://www.biology-online.org/kb/article.php?p=/2/8_mutations.htm (accessed 2010-2014).
33 Adapted from P. Schuster, 'Evolution and Design: A Review of the State of the Art in the Theory of Evolution', in *Creation and Evolution*, eds. S.O. Horn and S. Wiedenhofer, trans. M.J. Miller, San Francisco, Ignatius Press, 2007, p. 60.

Most importantly, we do not know, with scientific accuracy, if the sufficient elements in nature that have brought about the unbroken genealogical continuity in evolution that has been proposed actually happened. There are, in brief, epistemological gaps which prevent natural science from saying that a detailed theory of biotic evolution has been proven.[34]

In summarizing a chapter reviewing the state of the art in relation to evolution, Prof. Peter Schuster, addressing an audience that included Pope Benedict, said:

> According to the current state of our knowledge, pre-biological and biological evolution, from the first molecules capable of multiplication to the human being, appears to be a whole. We recognize that it is a process that goes on according to natural laws and needs no external intervention. Furthermore the natural scientist at present is making not one single observation that could be explained compellingly only by the interference of a supernatural being, nor is one necessary for the extrapolation of our present knowledge to the interpretation of events in the past... The development from the Big Bang down to the human being and eventually farther seems to be a unified cosmic process.[35]

The work that has been done in molecular biology, physical anthropology, palaeontology and categorizing species by morphology has affirmed the process of evolution from different pathways congruently. Schuster writes that an important feature of the evolution of the biosphere is that all cells, from the simplest bacterial life forms to the most highly developed animals, including man, use almost exactly the same biochemical machinery. The metabolic equipment of the cell remains unchanged, once set in

---

34 Coyne, op. cit.
35 Schuster, op. cit., p. 58.

motion, and remains virtually unchanged to this day.³⁶ Molecular biology has established a common history for the different life forms. An organism as complex as the human eye is closely related and shares a common molecular origin with all forms of the eye that are to be found in animals. All known forms of the eye have closely related genes that control the development of the eye in very different organisms. They appear to have a common origin in a single light-sensitive molecule.³⁷

From either perspective, whether the world evolved or was made according to a master plan, the evidence is in favour of the differences of species evolving from what existed at that time rather than that, in the first instance, they came into being wholly developed. Biological evolution works not like an engineer who thinks up a new design then makes the complete machine with parts designed for the purpose, but rather like an engineer working with whatever parts he has at hand to make whatever is possible with those parts.³⁸

In an editorial, in the *New York Times* on 7 July 2005, the Archbishop of Vienna, Chistoph Cardinal Schönborn,³⁹ criticized certain "neo-Darwinian" theories as incompatible with Catholic teaching. He rejected what he described as claims to an unguided, unplanned process of random variation and natural selection and he asserted that neo-Darwinism and the multiverse hypothesis in cosmology were invented to avoid the overwhelming evidence for purpose and design found in modern science. He asserted that

---

36 Ibid., p. 53.
37 W.J. Gehring, 'The genetic control of eye development and its implications for the evolution of the various eye-types', *International Journal of Developmental Biology*, vol. 46, 2002, pp. 65-73.
38 Ibid., p. 54.
39 Christoph Cardinal Schönborn, 'Finding Design in Nature', *New York Times*, 7 July 2005, http://www.millerandlevine.com/km/evol/catholic/schonborn-NYTimes.html (accessed 2010-2014).

any system of thought that denies or seeks to explain away the overwhelming evidence for design in biology is ideology, not science.

In a more nuanced presentation, Fr Coyne argues that God made a universe that is so prolific with the possibilities for these processes to succeed that when we talk about how we came to be we have to take the nature of the universe into consideration. He argues that the interplay of chance, necessity and opportunity leads inevitably to life and intelligence.[40] In other words, God did not rely on chance as Cardinal Schönborn claims neo-Darwinian theories assert. When God created the universe He created matter which would evolve according to a set of natural laws and would inevitably generate greater complexity, leading ultimately to human beings made in His image and likeness.

The International Theological Commission in the document *Communion and Stewardship: Human Persons Created in the Image of God*[41] explains a compatibility between the Big Bang theory and a belief in creation being formed from nothing. The theory does not contradict the doctrine. Clearly Big Bang theory does not in fact exclude the possibility of an antecedent stage of matter. Rather, it can be noted that the theory appears to provide merely indirect support for the doctrine of creation from nothing and the latter can only be known by faith.

The Commission asserts what the Catholic tradition affirms, that God, as universal transcendental cause, is the cause not only of existence but also the cause of causes.

> God's action does not displace or supplant the activity
> of creaturely causes, but enables them to act according

---

40 Coyne, op. cit.
41 International Theological Commission, 'Communion and Stewardship: Human Persons Created in the Image of God', *The July 2004 Vatican Statement on Creation and Evolution*, http://www.philvaz.com/apologetics/p80.htm (accessed 2010-2014).

to their natures and, nonetheless, to bring about the ends he intends. In freely willing to create and conserve the universe, God wills to activate and to sustain in act all those secondary causes whose activity contributes to the unfolding of the natural order which he intends to produce. Through the activity of natural causes, God causes to arise those conditions required for the emergence and support of living organisms, and, furthermore, for their reproduction and differentiation. Although there is scientific debate about the degree of purposiveness or design operative and empirically observable in these developments, they have de facto favored the emergence and flourishing of life. Catholic theologians can see in such reasoning support for the affirmation entailed by faith in divine creation and divine providence. In the providential design of creation, the triune God intended not only to make a place for human beings in the universe but also, and ultimately, to make room for them in his own trinitarian life. Furthermore, operating as real, though secondary causes, human beings contribute to the reshaping and transformation of the universe.[42]

According to a Catholic understanding of divine causality, true contingency in the created order is not incompatible with a purposeful divine providence. Even the outcome of a truly contingent natural process can nonetheless fall within God's providential plan for creation. According to St. Thomas Aquinas:

> ... the effect of divine providence is not only that things should happen somehow, but that they should happen either by necessity or by contingency. Therefore, whatsoever divine providence ordains to happen infallibly and of necessity happens infallibly and of necessity; and that happens from contingency, which the divine providence conceives to happen from contingency.[43]

---
42 Ibid.
43 St Thomas Aquinas, *Summa Theologica I*, Q. 22, Art. 4.

From a Catholic perspective, neo-Darwinians, who propose random genetic variation and natural selection as evidence that the process of evolution is absolutely unguided, are straying beyond what can be demonstrated by science. Divine causality can be active in a process that is both contingent and guided.[44]

Any evolutionary mechanism that is contingent can only be contingent because God made it so. An unguided evolutionary process – one that falls outside the bounds of divine providence – simply cannot exist because as St Thomas expressed it, "... the causality of God, Who is the first agent, extends to all being, not only as to constituent principles of species, but also as to the individualizing principles....It necessarily follows that all things, inasmuch as they participate in existence, must likewise be subject to divine providence".[45]

This can be expressed simply. As mentioned previously, Einstein found the idea of God playing dice unbelievable. Though there may be chance happenings, the result could not be unknown to God. Einstein explained that:

> The scientific method can teach us nothing else beyond how facts are related to, and conditioned by, each other. The aspiration toward such objective knowledge belongs to the highest of which man is capable, and you will certainly not suspect me of wishing to belittle the achievements and the heroic efforts of man in this sphere. Yet it is equally clear that knowledge of what is does not open the door directly to what *should be*.[46]

The International Theological Commission states what Catholic theology affirms, that particular actions of God bring about effects that transcend the capacity of created causes which

---
44 International Theological Commission, op. cit.
45 Aquinas, *Summa Theologica I*, Q. 22, Art. 2
46 Albert Einstein, *Out of My Later Years*, N.Y.: Philosophical Library, 1950.

act according to their natures. The Commission rejects appeals to divine causality to account for genuinely causal, as distinct from merely explanatory, gaps. Divine agency should not be inserted to fill in the "gaps" in human scientific understanding (as this would give rise to the so-called "God of the Gaps").

The Commission affirms that:

> The structures of the world can be seen as open to non-disruptive divine action in directly causing events in the world. Catholic theology affirms that the emergence of the first members of the human species (whether as individuals or in populations) represents an event that is not susceptible of a purely natural explanation and which can appropriately be attributed to divine intervention. Acting indirectly through causal chains operating from the beginning of cosmic history, God prepared the way for what Pope John Paul II has called "an ontological leap...the moment of transition to the spiritual." While science can study these causal chains, it falls to theology to locate this account of the special creation of the human soul within the overarching plan of the triune God to share the communion of trinitarian life with human persons who are created out of nothing in the image and likeness of God, and who, in his name and according to his plan, exercise a creative stewardship and sovereignty over the physical universe.[47]

This explanation fits with Cardinal Newman's previous comment to the effect that ordinary reproduction and the creation by God of a human soul happens from the *accidental* meeting and marriage of two persons, or even from sinful intercourse. From what may be a chance event there follows the very definite decision by God to create a spiritual soul. The idea of spiritual souls originating by God's intervention when the first human

---

47 International Theological Commission, op. cit.

being evolved from natural processes is thus no more problematic than the ordinary coming to be of a human being through natural conception.

Thus the concept of evolution does not exclude the possibility of an intelligent creator who willed the universe into being and in doing so envisaged the creation of each one of us, and that each of us would have an immortal soul individually created by Him. It is consistent with the theory of evolution for us to envisage that each of us has been created for a purpose: we exist for the purpose of communion with God. It is consistent with an acceptance of evolution for us to believe that we and the world around us reflect an intelligent design which God envisaged would develop according to the laws of nature; laws that tend toward greater complexity through natural processes and result in the complexity we find in human beings.

Thus the Genesis account, as an historical record and chronology, may not be consistent with the evidence of science but its essential message, about why we exist and that we were created by God for a purpose, are matters that are outside the scope of science and the science does not contradict the essential truths of our faith in that respect.

That there are scientists, such as Stephen Gould, who insist on an episodic, totally contingent and, therefore, non-repeatable evolutionary process, which would exclude that faith based account,[48] does not make evolutionary theory in itself inconsistent with faith; a faith in the deliberate choice of the Creator to make a universe that would develop just as this universe has developed, including the development of human beings made in His image and likeness.

On the issue of evolution, the view that science and Christian faith are in direct conflict depends on both a fundamentalist

---

48 Stephen Jay Gould, *The Structure of Evolutionary Theory*, Cambridge, Belknap Press, 2002.

interpretation of Scripture, as a detailed history of humankind, and on a view of evolution that is entirely dependent on chance and contains no intrinsic design. The latter is not a scientific view based on evidence and it is certainly not implied by evolutionary theory itself.

It is interesting to note that the problem of literal interpretations of Genesis and claims about the age of the world, based on Scripture, were a problem long before Darwin and the theories of evolution. It is worth noting that St Augustine had recognized the problem of too literal an interpretation of Genesis when he wrote:

> It not infrequently happens that something about the earth, about the sky, about other elements of this world, about the motion and rotation or even the magnitude and distances of the stars, about definite eclipses of the sun and moon, about the passage of years and seasons, about the nature of animals, of fruits, of stones, and of other such things, may be known with the greatest certainty by reasoning or by experience, even by one who is not a Christian. It is too disgraceful and ruinous, though, and greatly to be avoided, that he [the non-Christian] should hear a Christian speaking so idiotically on these matters, and as if in accord with Christian writings, that he might say that he could scarcely keep from laughing when he saw how totally in error they are... In view of this and in keeping it in mind constantly while dealing with the book of Genesis, I have, insofar as I was able, explained in detail and set forth for consideration the meanings of obscure passages, taking care not to affirm rashly some one meaning to the prejudice of another and perhaps better explanation.[49]

---

49 St Augustine, *The Literal Meaning of Genesis*, op. cit., vol. 1, bks. 19-20, chapter 19.

It is a pity that the Pope Paul V and his advisers did not follow Augustine on this in relation to asserting doctrine over scientific observation.

What would seem to be crucial to an understanding of Scripture and creation, from a Christian perspective, is the belief that God created everything out of nothing; that He created an orderly universe (such that the universe is not a product of chance) and that He sustains everything in being (everything depends on God for existence).[50] These beliefs are consistent with the idea that God created matter and the laws of nature by which matter would evolve to form life and, eventually, rational human life in the divine image and likeness.

The doctrine of creation rejects deism, Gnosticism, emanationism, pantheism and monism. Each creature is free but each has been individually created by God and remains dependent upon him for sustainment. Deism is the view that creation is like a clock that God makes, sets in motion and thereafter has no involvement with it. The doctrine of creation insists that God is involved in sustaining creation and all creation remains dependent upon him. The Gnostics thought that the variety of species represented disunity and decay in the material world, but Scripture teaches us that all creation is good. Emanationism is the view that creation is in fact a part of God that has broken away from him. Pantheism is the view that God is in everything and everything is in God. Monism is the view that there is only one substance, one being, and that is God: everything else either does not exist or it is God.[51]

The doctrine of creation means that God created freely, not

---

[50] David McDonald, 'What is the Catholic Position on Creationism and Evolution?', http://www.davidmacd.com/catholic/catholic_creationism.htm (accessed 2010-2014).
[51] Christoph Cardinal Schönborn, *Chance or Purpose? Creation, Evolution, and a Rational Faith*, San Francisco, Ignatius Press, 2007, p. 48.

out of necessity, and out of nothing. It is not that He created out of matter and shaped it to form the universe, but rather He made it out of nothing. Creatures of all varieties were also created by Him and this creation is continuous and dependent upon Him. God continues to guide the process of creation. All creation is good.

3
EVOLUTION AND THE HUMAN SOUL

3.1 Introduction

Darwin was not the first biologist to propose a theory that species evolved from other species.

In fact the idea of one creature coming from another creature was debated before the era of modern biology. St Augustine discussed what he called "traducianism" and was at least open to the idea of the human soul being generated by parents, rather than being individually created, saying, "I am more willing to continue listening to arguments on both sides than to establish one of the two theories at this time."[52]

St Thomas Aquinas very firmly rejected the idea:

> Regarding this question various opinions were expressed in antiquity. Some held that the soul of a child is produced by the soul of the parent just as the body is generated by the parent-body. Others maintained that all souls are created apart, moreover that they are united with their respective bodies, either by their own volition or by the command and action of God. Others again, declared that the soul in the moment of its creation is infused into the body. Though for a time these several views were upheld, and though it was doubtful which came nearest the truth (as appears from Augustine's commentary on Genesis 10, and from his books on the origin of the soul), the Church

---
[52] St Augustine, *The Literal Meaning of Genesis*, op. cit., vol. 2, bk. 10, chapter 20, p.123.

subsequently condemned the first two and approved the third.[53]

The issue of the evolution of the human soul is an obvious difficulty when trying to make a theory of evolution compatible with the Christian tradition and Holy Scripture. If human beings evolved and if the soul is the form of the body, how did the human body evolve and not the soul? We will return to these issues later.

In the modern era of biology, prior to Darwin's era, a Swedish botanist, Karl von Linné (1707-1778), developed a logical classification system for all living things which he proposed in his book *Systema Naturae*, which was first published in 1735. He classified these things by their genus. He did this by describing plants and animals on the basis of physical appearance and method of reproduction and he classified them relative to each other, according to the degree of their similarities. He was not the first to use the genus/species distinction. This is attributed to John Ray (1627-1705), an English naturalist. Controversially, for his time, this involved placing humans in the same genus as the other primates. It was controversial because it implied that human beings are animals. However this was nothing new to Christianity; both Boethius and St Thomas Aquinas had referred to human beings as rational animals. Erasmus Darwin, grandfather of Charles, also believed in evolution though he lacked a firm theory to explain how it could occur.[54]

Jean-Baptiste Chevalier de Lamarck (1744-1827) proposed a theory about these processes which proved to be incorrect. He believed that evolution was mostly due to the inheritance of acquired characteristics which formed as creatures adapted to their environments. Lamarck believed that microscopic organisms

---

53 Aquinas, *De Potentiâ*, Q 3, Art. 9.
54 Dennis O'Neill, 'Pre-Darwinian Theories', *Early Theories of Evolution*, http://anthro.palomar.edu/evolve/evolve_1.htm, (accessed 3 May 2011).

appear spontaneously from inanimate materials and then transmute, or evolve, gradually and progressively into more complex forms through a constant striving for perfection. The ultimate product of this goal-oriented evolution was thought by Lamarck to be humans.[55] This idea of adaptation is like believing that a giraffe could develop a longer neck to reach higher into the trees for food. It contrasts with the theory of natural selection in which it is those, with a slight advantage, who survive to breed with others with an advantage and thus bring about gradual advantageous change. It is worth noting that, in more recent times, science has accepted that the environment can cause genetic and epigenetic change. We see this occur harmfully when a cancer develops. However, it may be possible that such changes may be advantageous so that an individual thus adapts to the environment. So Lamarck was not totally wrong; the limited change that occurs and the fact that mostly it is not advantageous still requires natural selection to account for the fact that evolution progresses toward greater complexity and functionality. However to be part of evolution Lamarckian change needs to be inheritable and to be inheritable it needs to be genetic or epigenetic. There is some evidence that epigenetic change is inheritable. A couple who have no family history of obesity for instance, may, by being obese through lifestyle factors at the time a child is conceived, have caused the child to inherit the epigenetic changes that their own bodies had experienced. That would be a case of Lamarckian change which could lead, through natural selection, to the extinction of their own line.

3.2 Science and Compatibility with Scripture

In seeking a rapprochement between biology and Scripture it is important to note that an historical reading of Scripture, as though the Old Testament could be separated from the role of Christ and

---
[55] Ibid.

redemption, is in reality not Christian because it does not accept Scripture as an account of the relationship between God and man and the essential place that Jesus plays in it. A purely historical account would instead see it as a history of the peoples and their beliefs. The Early Fathers did not read the Old Testament, and Genesis in particular, with the belief that the world was indeed created in six days or that Genesis was literally true. They understood the Old Testament as having meaning in the light of the New Testament. Sin, original sin and the Fall only make sense in the light of Redemption. Even Jewish interpretation was not necessarily, or not even, literal and historicist. This was clear in the 19th century when Jewish writers such as Hermann Cohen, Franz Rosenzweig, Leo Strauss, and Isaac Breuer prevailed.[56] In a way they were writing in the tradition of the Alexandrian philosopher, Philo Judæus, who pursued the idea that Genesis was not so much a history of primal man but a symbol of the religious and moral development of the human soul.[57]

The historicism of contemporary fundamentalists appears as something of a reaction to contemporary evolutionism rather than adequately representing Christianity from its early sources until the present day. It is then seized upon by fundamentalist evolutionists to create a false dichotomy with religious belief by claiming that one must either accept science or accept religion but not both. In this way contemporaries such as Richard Dawkins[58] and Stephen Hawking[59] have adopted historicism as essential to Christianity.

In *The God Delusion*, Dawkins argues for competing views between science and religion. He argues that religious belief

---

56 D.N. Myers, *Resisting History: Historicism and Its Discontents in German-Jewish Thought*, Princeton, Princeton University Press, 2011.
57 'Philo Judæus', *Jewish Encyclopedia*, 1906, http://www.jewishencyclopedia.com/view.jsp?artid=281&letter=P#ixzz1LN6CLUdW, (accessed 3 May 2011).
58 Richard Dawkins, *The God Delusion*, Boston, Houghton Mifflin, 2006.
59 Stephen Hawking, *A Brief History of Time*, Bantam Books, 1988.

holds the view that the complexity of what we find in nature and in ourselves requires a designer, a complex being, to account for the complexity that we see. On the other hand science, through its understanding of evolution and the evidence that has established the theory of evolution, explains how from simple origins and principles something more complex can emerge via the processes of mutation and natural selection in the context of a battle for survival. He argues that science has shown that we do not need a God in order to be able to explain the complexity of the natural world.[60] He concludes:

> The temptation to attribute the appearance of a design to actual design itself is a false one, because the designer hypothesis immediately raises the larger problem of who designed the designer. The whole problem we started out with was the problem of explaining statistical improbability. It is obviously no solution to postulate something even more improbable.[61]

This is an application of Occam's razor, the principle that if one has two explanations for the same phenomenon then one should adopt the simpler of the two. Otherwise much of what Dawkins writes on this topic is a diatribe against the evils of religion and not really noteworthy because it is unbalanced: he presents a picture of God as a bully that is unrecognizable to most religious believers and unbalanced in relation to the history of Christianity. The Christian belief is in a God who loves us. Though evil has been done in the name of Christianity, this is neither characteristic of Christianity in the main nor a result of truly Christian belief.

The Dawkins argument, that the complexity of the universe is explicable by the theory of evolution, proposes a simpler alternative to what is often called Aquinas's teleological argument in which

---

60 Dawkins, op. cit.
61 Ibid. p. 158.

the latter argued that because things in the natural world clearly have a purpose there must be some intelligent being by whom all natural things are directed to their end.[62] This is to say, Dawkins suggests, that evolution provides a less complex explanation for why creatures in the natural world appear to have a purpose.

A simple response to Dawkins is to say the complexity may be explained by evolution but, however strong the evidence that creatures evolved, that does not disprove the need for a creator, who as the prime mover or first cause of the universe, set in place the matter and the capacity within it for more complex beings to evolve from lower orders of being. That is to say, one could invoke the other four explanations that Aquinas developed for the existence of God: the argument from motion, the argument from efficient causes, the argument from possibility and necessity; and the argument from the gradation of beings.[63]

An important point to make, in relation to claims that there is a conflict between religion and science regarding evolution, is that the claims are based on a literal reading of Scripture. The theory of evolution does not exclude the possibility that there is a creator. The argument is about how that creation was achieved in the first instance and how the creation of each individual human being is achieved. Trying to understand evolution is no more difficult than trying to understand the generation of each human life. The latter raises profound questions about the nature of the human soul and whether each human soul is individually created by God.

Science has given us an explanation of the formation of a new cell with a unique genetic identity partially inherited from each parent, and the role of that new human genome in the formation of that developing individual. That suggests what Augustine referred to as "traducianism" with the new body and soul coming from

---

62 Aquinas, *Summa Theologica I*, Q. 2, Art. 3.
63 Ibid.

the parents, rather than the new soul being specially created at conception. However, the emergence of the human body from sexual reproduction does not exclude a simultaneous creation of an immortal soul to which we can attribute the combined bodily and spiritual unity of the human person. Conceptually the most challenging aspect of this is the doctrinal claim made at Vienne that the soul forms and informs the matter[64] – that is to say, the soul is causally responsible for the human body and thus the person's existence as a material being. It is tempting to link the genome (the information source for the nature of the being, its genus and species) to the immortal soul of the person. But the genome, which is material, cannot be the human soul, which is immaterial. There is empirical evidence for the genome but there can be no empirical evidence for the soul. At best, the doctrine would allow us to propose that the genome is an instantiation or physical manifestation of the effects of the immortal soul. One of the most troubling or most unexplained phenomena is the phenomenon of consciousness. So far it has not been explained empirically and it is not observable. During my work chairing the Australian Government's committee of public enquiry into the unresponsive state, we were advised by those expert in the neurological sciences, that consciousness is an inference from a person's behaviour and not in itself observable.[65] If a person has some brain function it appears not to be possible to say categorically that he or she is unconscious. At the most it may be concluded that in the absence of responsiveness assessed by the systems of observation available there is no demonstration of consciousness.

Catholics, though not all Christians, presume, at least in their

---

[64] Council of Vienne, 1311-1312, *First Decree*, available at http://www.papalencyclicals.net/Councils/ecum15.htm#can1 (accessed 9 June 2011).

[65] National Health and Medical Research Council, *Ethical Guidelines for the Care of People in Unresponsiveness (Vegetative State) or a Minimally Responsive State*, Australian Government, 2008.

prayers, that an intelligent entity continues to be after death and prior to resurrection of the body, for we pray for that entity to intervene for us. The Council of Vienne was seemingly silent about the Scripture account of Jesus visiting the Holy Souls in purgatory between His death and resurrection. Was this wholly a spiritual visitation? Who was Jesus in that case, if not at that moment incarnated?

Followers of Karl Barth tend to believe instead that the soul dies with the body, awaiting resurrection.[66] That takes some explaining of Scripture. Some, such as Martin Luther, insist that Jesus did so not as a soul separated from the body, but as body and soul:

> ... I must not divide [the person of Christ] here either, but believe and say that the same Christ, God and man in one person, descended into hell but did not remain in it; as *Ps. 16:10* says of Him ... By the word "soul," He, in accordance with the language of the Scripture, does not mean, as we do, a being separated from the body, but the entire man, the Holy One of God, as He here calls Himself. But how it may have occurred that the man lies there in the grave, and yet descends into hell – that, indeed, we shall and must leave unexplained and uncomprehended; for ... we can only paint and conceive it in a coarse and bodily way and speak of it in pictures ...[67]

The scriptural passages upon which this teaching, which is regularly repeated by Christians in the Apostles' Creed, should be closely studied include: Job 38:17, Psalm 68:18-22; Matthew 12:38-41; Acts 2:22-32; Romans 10:7; Ephesians 4:7-10; 1 Peter 3:18-20, and 1 Peter 4:6.

---

66 Karl Barth, G.W. Bromiley and T.F. Torrance, *Church Dogmatics*, vol. 3, pt. 2, New York, T&T Clark, 1960, p. 370.

67 Martin Luther, sermon at Torgau in 1533, in *Historical Introductions to the Lutheran Confessions*, ed. F. Bente, retrieved from http://bookofconcord.org/historical-19.php (accessed 3 August 2012).

St Peter's first letter records:

> For Christ also suffered once for sins, the righteous for the unrighteous, to bring you to God. He was put to death in the body but made alive in the Spirit. After being made alive, he went and made proclamation to the imprisoned spirits –to those who were disobedient long ago when God waited patiently in the days of Noah while the ark was being built. In it only a few people, eight in all, were saved through water, and this water symbolizes baptism that now saves you also – not the removal of dirt from the body but the pledge of a clear conscience toward God. It saves you by the resurrection of Jesus Christ, who has gone into heaven and is at God's right hand – with angels, authorities and powers in submission to him.[68]

The *Catechism of the Catholic Church* states:

> Jesus "descended into the lower parts of the earth. He who descended is he who also ascended far above all the heavens." The Apostles' Creed confesses in the same article Christ's descent into hell and his Resurrection from the dead on the third day, because in his Passover it was precisely out of the depths of death that he made life spring forth ...[69]

This would seem to imply that the resurrection of the body followed after the descent into hell. I leave the interpretation of these passages to others who can study these texts in the biblical languages with much greater understanding than I can. However, I am inclined to accept the mystery of this event in the terms in which the words describe it.

The Catholic notion of a continued presence to whom one

---

68 1 Peter 3:18-22
69 *Catechism of the Catholic Church*, n. 631.

can continue to relate also appears to be very comforting.[70] The life of one's beloved is merely changed not ended. To a large extent the *spiritual dimensions* of death and conception remain a mystery. Science cannot provide an empirical answer. Scripture and Tradition have yielded partial answers that science can neither prove nor disprove.

3.3 Darwin's Theory

Darwin did not see a conflict between creationism and evolution. He writes:

> Authors of the highest eminence seem to be fully satisfied with the view that each species has been independently created. To my mind it accords better with what we know of the laws impressed on matter by the Creator, that the production and extinction of the past and present inhabitants of the world should have been due to secondary causes, like those determining the birth and death of the individual. When I view all beings not as special creations, but as the lineal descendants of some few beings which lived long before the first bed of the Silurian system was deposited, they seem to me to become ennobled. Judging from the past, we may safely infer that not one living species will transmit its unaltered likeness to a distant futurity. And of the species now living very few will transmit progeny of any kind to a far distant futurity; for the manner in which all organic beings are grouped, shows that the greater number of species of each genus, and all the species of many genera, have left no descendants, but have become utterly extinct.[71]

---

70 This difference between Catholic and Protestant belief about the soul at death and at resurrection is discussed in *About Bioethics Volume III: Transplantation, Biobanks and the Human Body*, Ballan, Connor Court, 2012, pp. 153 ff.

71 Charles Darwin, in 1859, *The Origin of the Species by Means of Natural Selection: The descent of man and selection in relation to sex*, repub. by *Encyclopaedia Britannica*, 1952, chapter 14.

This passage is interesting for it shows that Darwin did not claim, as modern evolution theory fundamentalists are want to claim, that evolution and belief in creation are incompatible. Darwin envisaged creation of life forms, from which even more complex forms of life would develop, by the accrual of very small changes from one generation to another and by the effects of natural selection, causing those with advantageous change to survive and therefore reproduce in greater proportions. He noted the creation of laws of nature that would make this happen. This seemed more marvellous to him than the immediate creation of the diversity that we see and the suitability of some species being more obviously adapted to their environments than others. Persons with dark skin in warmer climes compared to persons with white skin in colder climes is but one example.

He remarks:

> It is interesting to contemplate an entangled bank, clothed with many plants of many kinds, with birds singing on the bushes, with various insects flitting about, and with worms crawling through the damp earth, and to reflect that these elaborately constructed forms, so different from each other, and dependent on each other in so complex a manner, have all been produced by laws acting around us. These laws, taken in the largest sense, being Growth with Reproduction; inheritance which is almost implied by reproduction; Variability from the indirect and direct action of the external conditions of life, and from use and disuse; a Ratio of Increase so high as to lead to a Struggle for Life, and as a consequence to Natural Selection, entailing Divergence of Character and the Extinction of less-improved forms. Thus, from the war of nature, from famine and death, the most exalted object which we are capable of conceiving, namely, the production of the higher animals, directly follows. There is grandeur

in this view of life, with its several powers, having been originally breathed into a few forms or into one; and that, whilst this planet has gone cycling on according to the fixed law of gravity, from so simple a beginning endless forms most beautiful and most wonderful have been, and are being, evolved.[72]

Key to Darwin's theory of evolution is the fact that most species reproduce themselves in greater numbers than replacement requires. Survival of their species is a function of their relative capacities in competition with others to live and reproduce. It is this battle for survival that produces optimization of characteristics from one generation to another so that beings tend toward greater complexity.

It is important to note that the genetics that we take for granted and the molecular biology that now explains what Mendel observed were not available to Darwin.

The 19th century Austrian Augustinian monk, Gregor Johann Mendel, was a scientist and a mathematician. His application of mathematical principles to what he observed in breeding plants gained him fame as the figurehead of the new science of genetics.[73]

Darwin understood the changes that occurred between offspring and their parents in a quite different way. Mendel, as a mathematical genius, had identified the idea of a gene and even the idea of pairs of genes and alleles. He understood that in the process of pollination or fertilization there had to be a process in which some genes from each parent were not passed to the offspring; and so that, in reality, no individual passes his or her genetic inheritance completely on to an offspring. In the natural

---

72 Ibid.
73 Robin Marantz Henig, *Monk in the Garden: The Lost and Found Genius of Gregor Mendel, the Father of Genetics*, New York, Houghton Mifflin, 2000.

world parents who reproduce sexually are never cloned.[74] Their offspring share only some of the genes of each parent. The process of sexual reproduction almost always involves a selection of those genes which will be matched with their alleles (matched pairs) from the other parent in order to form a unique individual. The exceptions include the trisomy and monosomy disorders which involve a change in the pairing of the alleles.

Darwin appears not to have had a concept of a gene, as Mendel understood it, as a packet of genetic information. From observation, he knew that offspring took on inherited characteristics from both parents but he had no explanation for how that happened, or for the enormous variation that occurred between siblings of the same parents.

In fact, what we now know of molecular biology provides us with a greater understanding of the way in which inheritance can be affected by genetic change, in a single gene, during the process of reproduction.

Darwin's theory proceeds from three fairly simple observations:

- in the reproduction of living things, characteristics of the parents are transmitted to the offspring;
- the organisms in the population are not all identical, in other words there is a natural variation of their characteristics; and
- in every ecosystem many more offspring are produced than can survive on the basis of the available resources.

Darwin believed that the variability is caused by continuous and immeasurable minute changes that can arise as a consequence of a not entirely perfect process of reproduction. From these

---

[74] Note that "natural cloning", such as happens with the formation of monozygotic (identical) twins, is a form of asexual "parenting" though they are also siblings. The terminology becomes puzzling.

observations, he was led to conclude that those small changes produced characteristics that gave some advantage in terms of survival over generations and have a reinforcing effect on the proportions of individuals who have that change. So a small change may make little difference in one generation but if it gives some small advantage for survival then over a significant passage of time over, say for instance 100 years, the proportion of those with that advantage will outweigh the proportion who lacked the advantage. Thus, for Darwin, the theory of natural selection did not involve abrupt change in any one generation. It was all very gradual and the changes in any one generation were likely to be very minor and relatively insignificant.

Darwin's ideas of heredity were completely wrong. He believed in the heredity of acquired characteristics and did not distinguish between the germline and somatic cells. The understanding of meiosis and mitosis came later. In *The Origin of the Species* he assumed that inherited traits blended unevenly. The idea of genes or units of inheritance was unknown to him. The knowledge that we gained from Mendel's work allowed us to understand that there can be two different sorts of changes in genotype between parents and offspring:

- the hereditary units are recombined in different ways, thus resulting in new combinations with new characteristics for the carrier; and
- changes are introduced in the individual units and genuinely new alternative forms are generated.[75]

3.4 Genetics and Evolution

Since the time of Darwin, of course, evolutionary theory has undergone significant change, particularly in our understanding of

---

75 Schuster, op. cit., pp. 27-60.

molecular biology which can explain the nature of mutation in a way that Darwin simply could not have understood.

Crucial to understanding contemporary theories of evolution is the concept of genetic change or mutation. This happens far more frequently than many people often think, not only in gamete and embryo formation, but within the same individual as they develop.

There are several ways in which reproductive genetic variation is thought to occur including mutation, migration, genetic drift and natural selection which are included in the following explanations:

Mutation

A mutation involves a permanent change in the DNA sequence that makes up a gene. Some examples that we see are diseases like Downs Syndrome, Edwards Syndrome and Tay Sac's Disease. They are inherited from the parents but occur in the parental generation as a change in the gametes.

Migration

The movement of individuals to become part of a different population can introduce a change in that population.

Genetic drift

Some individuals do not to survive to reproduce because of chance. These chance changes from generation to generation are known as genetic drift.

Natural selection

Some features lead some individuals to have survival advantages over others. This may be related to changes in the environment. Overtime the process of breeding between those who have these advantages will lead to change in the population.

Macroevolution emphasizes the appearance of new,

physically distinct life forms that can be grouped with life forms of similar appearance in a taxonomic hierarchy.

Microevolution refers to genetic change within a single population: a population being defined by interbreeding.

Speciation

Species can be catalogued in two different ways:

- **Morphological species concept:** Oak trees look like oak trees, tigers will look like tigers. Morphology refers to the form and structure of an organism or any of its parts. The morphological species concept supports the widely held view that "members of a species are individuals that look similar to one another." This school of thought was the basis for Linneaus's original classification which is still broadly accepted and applicable today.[76]

- **Biological species concept:** This concept states that "a species is a group of actually or potentially interbreeding individuals who are reproductively isolated from other such groups."[77]

3.5 Molecular Biology and Evolution

The addition of molecular biology to evolutionary theory introduced some important elements in relation to the understanding of mutation:

- mutations or incidence of recombination are undirected, which means they do not occur more frequently just because their carrier has an advantage nor less often if they are detrimental to the carrier;
- it appears that the expediency of changes and

---

[76] University of Michigan, 'The Process of Speciation', *Introduction to Global Change*, 2002, http://www.globalchange.umich.edu/globalchange1/current/lectures/speciation/speciation.html (accessed 2010-2014).
[77] Ibid.

adaptations can be substantiated only *a posteriori* or as a consequence of optimization through variation and natural selection.[78]

This did away with such ideas as giraffes developing longer necks because this would give them an advantage in being able to reach the trees. In the first instance the changes that occurred are understood to be undirected by circumstances. For some reason a mutation in the genes would lead to a giraffe or some giraffes having a longer neck. In the process of reproduction and with the elapse of significant time, giraffes with a longer neck thus would have some advantage for their survival to reproduce and thus would survive in greater proportions than others; in the long-term, the others may even become extinct if the environmental circumstances are so challenging that only those with longer necks are able to survive. Thus the process of mutation and natural selection produces significant change. Darwin's theory held that this kind of change in the species is very gradual but contemporary molecular biology accepts that the effect of a single mutation could in fact be more dramatic. Therefore the change in population could happen more rapidly following a significant mutation that gave advantage to the carrier.

In the process of duplication of a cell, transcription errors can occur. That is to say that copying errors occur; what is being copied in cell duplication is a sequence of nucleic acids and it is their order, within the molecule, that determines the gene. Also within the cell are epigenetic mechanisms. The functions of a cell are determined in part by the genes within the cell, that is the order of nucleic acids, but there is also a function which determines the way in which they are read, which genes may be read and which genes ignored. So in a human being, usually, the somatic cells all have the same genetic coding but the cells differentiate

---

[78] Schuster, op. cit.

from their early embryonic cells to form all the different types of cells that we find in different parts of the body, such as liver cells, heart muscle cells, brain cells and so on. Those differences are not differences in the genetic code of the cells, rather they are differences in the epigenetic mechanisms in the different types of cell. Changes in the copying of those epigenetic mechanisms can also cause mutation when those differences affect the germ cells and are inherited by the offspring. Thus offspring may inherit a new characteristic possessed by neither parent. Presumably just such a mutation or mutations would have resulted in a human being conceived by non-human parents.

In the evolution versus creation debate much attention is given to the notion of chance. Some argue that the evolution of one species into another depends on random chance. We tend to describe something as happening from chance when we do not understand what might have caused the change. Mutations are infrequent, but not so when looked at in the time frame that is applied to evolution. Some kinds of mutation are more frequent than others. For instance, Downs Syndrome happens in approximately one in 300 pregnancies and one in 800 births[79] and Edwards Syndrome one in 3000 pregnancies and one in 5000 births.[80] The biological processes that result in growth and reproduction are in fact quite efficient at doing so accurately. For most people mutation is not a factor in their having been conceived but for the purposes of evolution a rate of one in a few thousand would be more than adequate. Mutations are few and far between, and most often

---

[79] Based on estimates by National Institute of Child Health & Human Development, 'Down syndrome rates', retrieved from http://web.archive.org/web/20060901004316/http://www.nichd.nih.gov/publications/pubs/downsyndrome/down.htm#Questions, (accessed 9 June 2011).

[80] Based on estimates in the USA, retrieved from Right Diagnosis website, 'Statistics about Edwards Syndrome', http://www.rightdiagnosis.com/e/edwards_syndrome/stats.htm#medical_stats, (accessed 9 June 2011).

not advantageous. This has led many to claim that evolution is impossible, or at least improbable, because the development of more and more complex beings would rely so heavily on mutations to produce changes and would therefore be unlikely because of the infrequency of mutations. The theory of evolution is not based just on randomness: it is based on natural selection and the elapse of large periods of time so that a very minor change, producing a minor advantage, can have a significant effect on the population over time. In other words, natural selection is not random: it is directed towards advantage and therefore greater complexity.

In giving accounts of evolution it is often postulated that the range of species that we now know may have come from a common source. This is often depicted as a tree of life with all the species branching off at different times in terms of their ancestors, until we get to the range of species that we now know shown as the twigs at the end of the branches of the tree; the intervening branches having been largely lost, leaving just the twigs. The fossil record shows us only glimpses of parts of the branches.

In Darwin's time these branches and twigs were described morphologically; scientists looked at the appearance of the functions of each species and postulated how one species may have developed from another, including the imagining of a species going from water dwelling to developing lungs, to becoming amphibious, to eventually walking on land and losing the capacity to survive underwater; and perhaps developing the ability to fly as well.

Since the advent of molecular biology, these depictions were more likely to be drawn to explain the molecular changes that differentiate one species from another. Scientists have been able to identify the similarities that occur between species, with similar genes having similar functions across species, indicating a shared ancestry of a mutation that produced the particular gene in the first instance and gave the creature that had it an advantage. So we now have molecular genetic family-trees of life forms. What may be surprising is that there appears to be a close correlation between the old morphological family trees based on appearance and function, and the more contemporary molecular genetic family-trees based on genetic similarities.

The circumstances of temperature, oxygen and water availability that allowed life to develop on this planet are an extraordinary combination of events, perhaps more mysterious in their coinciding than the evolutionary process which we have been discussing. That raises an interesting question as to whether it was directed or whether it was simply chance that from all the immense universe it happened to be the case that the circumstances in which life could develop occurred on this planet. The immensity of the universe adds some numerical credence to the possibility of life occurring somewhere, and as it happens, on Earth.

Evolutionary theory is, as we have seen, based on the idea that chance events lead to changes that are reproduced in the development of a being – either from the parents in the case of sexual reproduction or asexually, from a single parent, in the case of lower organisms such as amoeba and earthworms – combined with the mechanism of natural selection that causes optimal change to survive, to be reproduced and to increase in proportion. The theory holds that the immense complexity of a human being could have been developed from very humble origins in the Big Bang or some such start to the universe. Of course, from a divine perspective all that would have been foreseen in whatever act of creation it was that began the universe and the physical rules of nature by which it is governed.

Often in the language that is used, atheist biologists make mistakes and attribute purpose to the functions that they see. However that cannot be the reality for an atheistic evolutionary theory. In such a theory nothing comes to be for a purpose. Rather things come to be by chance and then are subjected to an optimization process that keeps them in existence if they give the creature a survival advantage. In a sense survival of genes becomes the teleology of evolutionary theory. This was postulated by Richard Dawkins in his book *The Selfish Gene*.[81] However survival in this scenario is not a conscious purpose. This lack of purpose or design is part of the challenge to religion, which sees all creation as being a result of a divine decision to design and create. In other words, religion sees all creation as purposive. The difficulty for us is to reconcile the biological processes, which are the basis of evolution, with the role and function of a divine Creator. In evolutionary theory, one of the most challenging events for us is the implication that somewhere, at some time, an animal gave birth to a human being with an immortal soul. This raises the question as to whether we see all of creation as having been created by God with evolution as part of the design and plan, or whether we see the Creator as intervening at the point when evolution reaches the pinnacle of developing a being who has rationality and who is then made *imago Dei* by the infusion of an immortal soul.

In presenting Darwin's theory of evolution and its affirmation by contemporary science, I do not want to give the impression that there are no questions unanswered and that there may not be new developments which challenge the tendency of contemporary theory on the process of natural selection. The combination of chance, on the one hand, and the mechanism of natural selection, on the other, provide a very simple explanation for the growing complexity which leads from the simplest of all creatures to the complexity of a human being over a long period of time; at the same time that complexity contains incredible evidence

---

[81] Richard Dawkins, *The Selfish Gene*, New York, Oxford, 1976.

of purposiveness and design. The two concepts of chance and mechanism are not themselves beyond analysis.

In his discussion of chance, Father Paul Erbrich[82] points out that, in evolutionary biology, chance has come to mean arbitrary, and certainly excludes purpose or design. The concept of a mechanism in natural selection understood as a happening that comes about through change, which produces an advantage in a competitive environment, excludes the possibility of any kind of adaptation by a creature or its species itself. Evidence of a creature producing inheritable change in response to its own environment would be challenging for evolutionary theory. Larmarckian evolution is not impossible. There just seems to be little evidence for it.[83] There are also questions about whether natural selection in itself, and alone, is sufficient because there seems to be so much in the environment, which has desirable qualities, that has nothing to do seemingly with survival advantage. In looking at the beauty of a mountain range or a sunset it is difficult to explain how it is beautiful and that we are able to observe its beauty. By what mechanism could those things have been selected for survival advantage? Is it simply that the mountain is beautiful, we are able to observe it and these are the coincidental results of change and survival advantage?

3.6 Evolution and the Soul

One theologian who embraced the theory of evolution very strongly, including the evolution of the soul, was Fr. Pierre Teilhard de Chardin. It is possible, perhaps even likely, that the encyclical *Humani Generis*[84] was addressed to the teaching of de

---

[82] Paul Erbrich, 'The Problem of Creation and Evolution', in S.O. Horn et al, *Creation and Evolution*, Ignatius Press, 2006, pp. 70-83.

[83] Note that we are familiar with one kind of Lamarckian adaptation: the ability of the immune system to adapt and change so as to develop resistance to infection. We know also that that resistance can be passed from mother to child.

[84] Pope Pius XII, op. cit.

Chardin. Teilhard de Chardin accepted that humans, being body and soul, have evolved; he held that humanity was just at a stage of evolution moving towards what he called the Omega, which in some of his writings refers to Christ according to the passage where John reports the Lord God as saying: "I am the Alpha and the Omega" (Rev 1:8).[85]

De Chardin rejects the idea of a world created fully formed. He rejects the notion of original sin which he considers to be a static event. In doing so, he rejects the idea that actual death is a result of original sin. Instead he holds that death was part of life before humankind evolved and so it cannot be the result of sin but it is the result of nature. In rejecting the concept of original sin he rejects the notion of expiation and reparation and, therefore, Christ's redemptive mission expressed in terms of liberating us from the effects of sin. He argues that in accepting evolution we must accept a radicalization of biblical understanding. He writes of consciousness evolving from matter but sees it as just a step on the way to an even higher level. He writes of Christ's redemption, in those terms, calling us to a unity of consciousness as we continue to evolve to a higher state, what he calls a super soul.[86]

In human reproduction a new cell comes to be, that has originated in the fusion of sperm and an egg from the respective parents. Within that cell there is an inherent capacity to cause the development of an embryo, to direct its own differentiation and growth in such a way as to form the complex being who arrives in the mother's arms following birth. It is very difficult not to see that growth and development as purposive. The generation of a human being in this way prompts the question: who or what brought about this capacity for internal organization? What happens between the

---

85 Pierre Teilhard de Chardin, *Christianity and Evolution*, trans. R. Hague, New York, Harcourt, 1971.
86 Ibid.

existence of that first cell and the birth of a child seems to have purpose and is not random. In this way all organisms seem to be purposive. On the other hand, evolutionary biologists would see this complexity as being the result of chance, change and of the optimization of the process of natural selection.

Clearly the difficulty for us is our belief that every single human being has an immortal soul, immediately created by God. Following the teaching of St Thomas, on the basis of which the Council of the Vienne proclaimed the nature of an immortal soul and its function in forming and informing the matter that constitutes the body, we have the idea that the human soul is created by a deliberate act of God and that the immortal soul directs the formation of the body and gives it its earthly temporal life. Catholics believe, further, that earthly temporal life ends when the soul separates from the body. In this Catholics differ from many Protestants who, following the teaching of Karl Barth, believe that the soul dies with the body and awaits the last day when the soul and body will be resurrected in glory.[87]

One way of understanding this is to consider that at some point, when the evolutionary process reached its pinnacle in the complex being that we recognize as a human being, God endowed that being with an immortal soul at the moment of its formation and continues to do so with each new fertilization, enabling the coming to be of a new cell with the capacity to develop to human adulthood.

An alternative way of looking at all of this is to see that, at the beginning of time, God created the universe in such a way that these processes of chance, change and the mechanism of optimization through natural selection were part of His plan. This plan included the function of the spiritual dimension in relation to each being having a soul formed according to that original plan and being meant to come into existence as an individual being. At some point,

---

[87] Barth, op. cit., p. 370.

that growing complexity resulted in a being with the capacity for doubting, wondering, reasoning and loving; an *imago Dei* with an immortal soul. Such a view would be compatible with the idea that the existence of every moment and every part of the universe is sustained by God's will. It is a view that would seem to be consistent with a loving God who loves us and wants us to love Him and who sets us free, rather than being a God who intervenes constantly.

In these alternatives, on the one hand, there is a God who intervenes to create an immortal soul for each individual when the biological events result in a being who has the inherent radical capacity for rationality, which the possession of a human genome causes and, on the other hand, a God who has created and sustains a universe in which human beings have evolved to the point where they have the form of the *imago Dei*. A problem with this latter view is that it would seem to imply the evolution of the soul.

A third view would have the biological material world existing independently of the spiritual world so that human beings would exist as a duality of soul and spirit. That is not Catholic tradition. The Council of Vienne is quite explicit about the unity of the soul and body and the causal role of the soul in forming and informing the matter of body. This makes the spiritual world relate to the material world in a dynamic causal relationship.

3.7 The Church and Evolution of the Human Soul

On 24 April 1870, eleven years after the publication of the *Origin of the Species*, the First Vatican Council, famous for proclaiming the doctrine of papal infallibility, addressed, in categorical terms, a number of ideas that were around at that time:

On God the creator of all things

1. If anyone denies the one true God, creator and lord of things visible and invisible: let him be **anathema**.

2. If anyone is so bold as to assert that there exists nothing besides matter: let him be **anathema**.

3. If anyone says that the substance or essence of God and that of all things are one and the same: let him be **anathema**.

4. If anyone says that finite things, both corporal and spiritual, or at any rate, spiritual, emanated from the divine substance; or that the divine essence, by the manifestation and evolution of itself becomes all things or, finally, that God is a universal or indefinite being which by self determination establishes the totality of things distinct in genera, species and individuals: let him be **anathema**.

5. If anyone does not confess that the world and all things which are contained in it, both spiritual and material, were produced, according to their whole substance, out of nothing by God; or holds that God did not create by his will free from all necessity, but as necessarily as he necessarily loves himself; or denies that the world was created for the glory of God: let him be **anathema**.[88]

None of these seem to touch directly on the question of evolution and whether the human soul may have evolved. However, Pope Pius XII, on 12 August 1950, would seem to have accepted the possibility of the evolution of the body, but not the evolution of the soul. In the encyclical *Humani Generis,* Pope Pius XII taught:

> For these reasons the Teaching Authority of the Church does not forbid that, in conformity with the present state of human sciences and sacred theology, research and discussions, on the part of men experienced in both fields, take place with regard to the doctrine of evolution, in as far as it inquires into the origin of the human body

---

[88] First Vatican Council. *Dogmatic Constitution on the Catholic Faith (Dei Filius),* (1869-1870), retrieved from http://www.catholicplanet.org/councils/20-Dei-Filius.htm (accessed 2010-2014).

as coming from pre-existent and living matter – for the Catholic faith obliges us to hold that souls are immediately created by God. However this must be done in such a way that the reasons for both opinions, that is, those favorable and those unfavorable to evolution, be weighed and judged with the necessary seriousness, moderation and measure, and provided that all are prepared to submit to the judgment of the Church, to whom Christ has given the mission of interpreting authentically the Sacred Scriptures and of defending the dogmas of faithful. Some however rashly transgress this liberty of discussion, when they act as if the origin of the human body from pre-existing and living matter were already completely certain and proved by the facts which have been discovered up to now and by reasoning on those facts, and as if there were nothing in the sources of divine revelation which demands the greatest moderation and caution in this question.[89]

This passage implies an acceptance of the possibility of the evolution of the body but rejects the idea that the soul might have evolved. The word "creari" means create, bring into being, make, procreate, beget, sire, produce, bear, bring about, give birth to, produce fruit, cause to grow, elect, appoint, invest, institute, conjure

---

[89] Pope Pius XII, op. cit., from the Latin: "Quamobrem Ecclesiae Magisterium non prohibet quominus « evolutionismi » doctrina, quatenus nempe de humani corporis origine inquirit ex iam exsistente ac vivente materia oriundi – animas enim a Deo immediate creari catholica fides non retinere iubet – pro hodierno humanarum disciplinarum et sacrae theologiae statu, investigationibus ac disputationibus peritorum in utroque campo hominum pertractetur ; ita quidem ut rationes utriusque opinionis, faventium nempe, vel obstantium, debita cum gravitate, moderatione ac temperantia perpendantur ac diiudicentur; dummodo omnes parati sint ad Ecclesiae iudicio obtemperandum, cui a Christo munus demandatum est et Sacras Scripturas authentice interpretandi et fidei dogmata tuendi . Hanc tamen disceptandi libertatem nonnulli temerario ausu transgrediuntur, cum ita sese gerant quasi si ipsa humani corporis origo ex iam exsistente ac vivente materia per indicia hucusque reperta ac per ratiocinia ex iisdem iudiciis deducta, iam certa omnino sit ac demonstrata; atque ex divinae revelationis fontibus nihil habeatur, quod in hac re maximam moderationem et cautelam exigat."

up. The word "immediate" means absolute, not mediated, next. In this context the phrase would seem to exclude the soul coming to be, in a universe of God's creation, through evolutionary processes that finally result in a being who has a rational nature and is *imago Dei* in possession of an immortal soul. The passage would seem to accept that the body may have evolved in that fashion but that the creation of the soul by God must be immediate. It would seem that the creation of a human being by God would not be immediate creation if it came about by God creating a universe which then evolved to produce human beings including their immortal souls. This requires an acceptance of one form of origin for the human body and another for the human soul. This is not to say necessarily that there are two beginnings nor that both origins are not from God. The account in Genesis 2 has God taking dust and breathing life into it; this could be taken as consistent with a lower life form mutating to form a higher life form into which God breathes eternal life.

The Congregation for the Doctrine of the Faith has a discussion about the nature of the human body in relation to the human soul. The congregation writes:

> For it is only in keeping with his true nature that the human person can achieve self-realization as a "unified totality": and this nature is at the same time corporal and spiritual. By virtue of its substantial union with a spiritual soul, the human body cannot be considered as a mere complex of tissues, organs and functions, nor can it be evaluated in the same way as the body of animals; rather it is a constitutive part of the person who manifests and expresses himself through it.[90]

---

[90] Congregation for the Doctrine of the Faith, *Donum Vitae*, English translation: *Instruction on Respect for Human Life in its Origin and on the Dignity of Procreation*, 22 February 1987.

Evolution and the Human Soul

And further:

> Certainly no experimental datum can be in itself sufficient to bring us to the recognition of a spiritual soul; nevertheless, the conclusions of science regarding the human embryo provide a valuable indication for discerning by the use of reason a personal presence at the moment of this first appearance of a human life: how could a human individual not be a human person? The Magisterium has not expressly committed itself to an affirmation of a philosophical nature, but it constantly reaffirms the moral condemnation of any kind of procured abortion. This teaching has not been changed and is unchangeable.[91]

The nature of the human soul and its origin in a human life are considered to be more matters of philosophical conjecture than matters of doctrine.

The Second Vatican Council made no direct mention of evolutionary theory that I have been able to find. However, Pope John Paul II addressed the above passage from Pope Pius XII in the following way:

> The Church's magisterium is directly concerned with the question of evolution, for it involves the conception of man: Revelation teaches us that he was created in the image and likeness of God (cf. Gn 1:27-29). The conciliar constitution *Gaudium et Spes* has magnificently explained this doctrine, which is pivotal to Christian thought. It recalled that man is "the only creature on earth that God has wanted for its own sake" (No. 24). In other terms, the human individual cannot be subordinated as a pure means or a pure instrument, either to the species or to society; he has value *per se*. He is a person. With his intellect and his will, he is capable of forming a relationship of commu-

---
[91] Ibid.

nion, solidarity and self-giving with his peers. St. Thomas observes that man's likeness to God resides especially in his speculative intellect, for his relationship with the object of his knowledge resembles God's relationship with what he has created (*Summa Theologica* I-II:3:5, ad 1). But even more, man is called to enter into a relationship of knowledge and love with God himself, a relationship which will find its complete fulfillment beyond time, in eternity. All the depth and grandeur of this vocation are revealed to us in the mystery of the risen Christ (cf. *Gaudium et Spes*, 22). It is by virtue of his spiritual soul that the whole person possesses such a dignity even in his body. Pius XII stressed this essential point: If the human body take its origin from pre-existent living matter, the spiritual soul is immediately created by God ("animas enim a Deo immediate creari catholica fides nos retinere iubei"; *Humani Generis*, 36). Consequently, theories of evolution which, in accordance with the philosophies inspiring them, consider the spirit as emerging from the forces of living matter or as a mere *epiphenomenon* of this matter, are incompatible with the truth about man. Nor are they able to ground the dignity of the person.[92]

A crucial issue in this is the teaching that the human person who "is the only creature on earth which God willed for itself, cannot fully find himself except through a sincere gift of himself."[93] What is clear, in our tradition, is that we are created by God, made to be loved by God and for us to love him. It is not clear to me why it is that we must insist on this creation being immediate, thus excluding the possibility of the soul and body evolving together, instead of seeing the body evolving and the soul being immediately created at the point that a new individual with a rational nature emerges.

---

92 Pope John Paul II, *Truth Cannot Contradict Truth*, op. cit.
93 Second Vatican Council, *Gaudium et Spes*, 7 December 1965, n. 24.

The latter would seem to involve an interventionist God rather than a God who creates the universe, sustains it and allows it to unfold, including giving complete free will to human beings when they emerge in that universe. The former seems a more attractive version of events than the idea of God intervening to create each individual life as it comes to be in the fusion of sperm and an egg. I guess that holding to the notion of an individual act of creation for each of us is a rejection of the idea that true freedom could emerge from matter and through the determinism we associate with the material world.[94] Would belief in the soul evolving from matter imply some kind of determinism in which everything could be attributed to the activities of molecules, seeing that molecules and their activities have clear lines of causation?

However, Pope John Paul II is quite clear in excluding the possibility that the soul may have evolved. This implies, then, the suggestion that at some point God creates an individual soul. This is not just an issue for evolution. The issue arises with the origin of every human being. We are familiar with the biological process by which a man and a woman unite in one flesh: through their union a sperm and an egg unite to form a new cell which has the capacity to develop to human adulthood and has the inherent capacity for rationality. On this account God would recognize this moment and a new soul would be created with every fertilization event. As I mentioned earlier, this is the doctrine that was firmly held by St Thomas Aquinas but which had been questioned by St Augustine.

We know from the science that what causes a human being to have the inherent capacity for rationality is the possession of a human genome. This is to say that what separates a human being from other animals is the particular nature of the structure and organism of molecules that form the human genome. Evolutionary theory has it that the genome has evolved through many stages

---

[94] I am grateful to Adam Cooper for this suggestion (9 June 2011).

of molecular change. This raises questions about the origin and function of the soul.

Understanding of the human soul first became doctrine at the Council of Vienne which taught, "In order that all may know the truth of the faith in its purity and all error may be excluded, we define that anyone who presumes henceforth to assert defend or hold stubbornly that the rational or intellectual soul is not the form of the human body of itself and essentially, is to be considered a heretic."[95]

This decree formed the following explanation:

> Adhering firmly to the foundation of the catholic faith, other than which, as the Apostle testifies, no one can lay, we openly profess with holy mother church that the only begotten Son of God, subsisting eternally together with the Father in everything in which God the Father exists, assumed in time in the womb of a virgin the parts of our nature united together, from which he himself true God became true man: namely the human, passible body and the intellectual or rational soul truly of itself and essentially informing the body. And that in this assumed nature the Word of God willed for the salvation of all not only to be nailed to the cross and to die on it, but also, having already breathed forth his spirit, permitted his side to be pierced by a lance, so that from the outflowing water and blood there might be formed the one, immaculate and holy virginal mother church, the bride of Christ, as from the side of the first man in his sleep Eve was fashioned as his wife, in this way, to the determinate figure of the first and old Adam, who according to the Apostle is a type of the one who was to come, the truth might correspond in our last Adam, that is to say in Christ.[96]

---
95 Council of Vienne, op. cit.
96 Ibid.

What we understand from science of the human genome must then be applied in the context of our understanding that we have a human, passible body and an intellectual or rational soul truly of itself and essentially informing the body. The teaching on evolution seems to require us to see the body and soul as having two different modes of generation in the one origin;[97] the body is created by God like all creation, but may have evolved from lower forms, but the soul is immediately created by God. The soul is that which forms or informs the matter that forms the body. Part of that matter is the human genome which must therefore be the result of a human soul. The genome must therefore be the causal agent by which the soul informs the matter that is the body.

This brings us back to the question of whether belief in individual creation by God in this way is compatible with science. It suggests that science deals exclusively with the natural world, that is the material world, and that the spiritual world exists outside of the world of evidence and is a matter of belief and truth known through Divine Revelation. This does not mean that there is no relationship between the physical world and the spiritual world. The Early Fathers believed that we could seek to understand more of the Creator by understanding the nature of His creation.

3.8 Evolution of the Soul

Father Pierre Teilhard de Chardin was referred to earlier. His account is problematic because he believed, contrary to the doctrine, that it was not just the human body that evolved but also the human soul. However an interesting aspect of his account is that he believed that human beings were just a stage of evolution and that obviously there were further stages to come. He saw Christ as the Omega. In other words he saw Christ as representing

---

[97] I am grateful to Adam Cooper for this suggestion (9 June 2011).

that toward which we were evolving. He saw us moving from inanimate matter to animate matter to conscious life. He wrote about us evolving to a state of having not just a soul but a super soul and in this he envisaged a level of higher consciousness and unity. For Teilhard de Chardin, the noosphere emerged through and is constituted by the interaction of human minds. The noosphere has grown in step with the organization of the human mass in relation to itself as it populates the earth. As mankind organizes itself in more complex social networks, the higher the noosphere will grow in awareness. It would be interesting to know what Teilhard de Chardin would have made of the development of the Internet. He clearly saw growing levels of communication between human beings as a development towards a higher state. Given what the Internet is used for and the proportion of it that is given over to pornography and other base developments, it is hard to see the Internet as representing a higher state of consciousness. It may reflect more consciousness and more communication but not at a higher level. If anything the communication is at a much lower level of banality. However it is true that we have almost immediate access to information and are seemingly much closer to events around the world and able to take greater responsibility both individually and as community in serving the needs of others. The images that provoke our sympathy and effective response are almost immediately with us wherever they occur.

His work does however raise the question, if we accept the concept of evolution, do we believe that human beings are the pinnacle of evolution and therefore there is to be no further evolution of human beings, or do we believe that we are evolving towards a being who is more complex? An interesting aspect of consciousness and reason is that human beings, it would seem to appear, have developed to a level where we can consciously interfere with the process of evolution. Evolution works on the basis of the battle for survival, the survival of the fittest and a process by which the more complex are more likely to have the advantage to survive. By our use of technology to treat illness, so that those who have illness may still be able to reproduce, and by our understanding of equality, in relation to disability and race, it would seem that we have interrupted the process of evolution by protecting those who would not have survived to reproduce otherwise. In fact one of the fears of the supporters of eugenics, such as Winston Churchill, is that the world would be overrun by the feeble-minded classes, because educated intelligent people have fewer children than those who are less educated and less able. He advocated the passing of the UK 1913 *Mental Deficiency Act* that provided for the compulsory sterilization of those in mental asylums.

> The unnatural and increasingly rapid growth of the feeble-minded classes, coupled with a steady restriction among all the thrifty, energetic and superior stocks constitute a race danger which it is impossible to exaggerate. I feel that the sources from which the stream of madness is fed should be cut off and sealed up before another year has passed.[98]

We practise eugenics via prenatal and preimplantation genetic diagnosis and even with infanticide, often by neglect after birth. To that extent, we are preventing the birth of those who would have survived with disabilities but we do not prevent their parents from reproducing and giving birth to carriers. Many of those who are eliminated because they had disabilities would not have been able to reproduce in any case. So it is not fear of the effects of those practices on future populations that drives modern eugenics. The effect is on the immediate population but not necessarily on

---

98 Winston Churchill to Prime Minister Asquith in 1910, as quoted by C. Ponting, *The Guardian Outlook*, 20 June 1992.

the populations to come. As discussed in a later chapter on the population question, we do know that the more educated the population is, the fewer children that population has. So if there is continuing evolution of the human population it would seem to be towards those populations that are less educated, if anything, but the reality would seem to be that, with the dawn of reason, the process of evolution would seem to have reached a finality in human beings.

Teilhard de Chardin's idea that Jesus is the pinnacle of the evolutionary process is obviously attractive; but the kind of evolution that is required for us to become more like Jesus would seem to be social and intellectual rather than biological. In our Christian understanding of the Incarnation he was a man, not a superman, even though he was also God. That he was also God does not change our belief that he was, as man, one of us.

4

IN THE BEGINNING ...

4.1 Creation Out Of Nothing

In this chapter we will explore the meaning of creation in revelation and the apostolic tradition. For as the Second Vatican Council expressed it:

> ... there exists a close connection and communication between sacred tradition and Sacred Scripture. For both of them, flowing from the same divine wellspring, in a certain way merge into a unity and tend toward the same end. For Sacred Scripture is the word of God inasmuch as it is consigned to writing under the inspiration of the divine Spirit, while sacred tradition takes the word of God entrusted by Christ the Lord and the Holy Spirit to the Apostles, and hands it on to their successors in its full purity, so that led by the light of the Spirit of truth, they may in proclaiming it preserve this word of God faithfully, explain it, and make it more widely known. Consequently it is not from Sacred Scripture alone that the Church draws her certainty about everything which has been revealed. Therefore both sacred tradition and Sacred Scripture are to be accepted and venerated with the same sense of loyalty and reverence.[99]

Far from being in opposition to science, Christian belief can actually be attributed with creating the circumstances in which science could prosper. As the former Cardinal Ratzinger, Pope

---
99 Second Vatican Council, *Dei Verbum*, 18 November 1965, n. 9.

Benedict explains in his reflections on Genesis 1-3 that through the Word of God human beings ceased to care about gods and demons and a world of chaotic forces. Christians believe in a God who acts through reason and love and not arbitrarily. This belief supported the world of science and the belief that every event has a cause. This liberated us from magic and superstition.

> The world was freed so that reason might lift itself up to God and so that human beings might approach this God fearlessly. In this Word they experienced the true enlightenment that does away with the gods and the mysterious powers and that reveals to them that there is only one power everywhere and that we are in his hands. This is the living God, and this same power (which created the earth and the stars and which bears the whole universe) is the very one whom we meet in the Word of Holy Scripture. In this Word we come into contact with the real primordial force of the world and with the power that is above all powers.[100]

As the Pope explained, in seeking to apply a scriptural account of creation we are not reading a scientific text and we need to distinguish between the form of portrayal and the content of what is portrayed. The form is taken from the knowledge of the time: the concepts and ideas of the time. What is crucial is the notion of creation.

That then poses the question, what does Christian faith believe about creation? Central to what we believe about creation is belief in creation out of nothing. This doctrine was defined very early in the life of the church.

The doctrine on the creation out of nothing seems to have been part of the development of the early church, probably around the third or fourth century, when the Scriptures were read

---

[100] Ratzinger, *'In the beginning ... '*, op. cit.

as an entirety. So the first two books of Genesis, that give us an account of the creation of the world and the creatures within it, were read alongside the gospel of John, "In the beginning was the Word ..."[101]

The Christian approach to creation was very different from the beliefs of the time which held that the universe was eternal and had no beginning. The questions that were pursued would have meant placing the universe on a par with God. Even the idea that God had created out of pre-existing formless matter was rejected. The Christian view was that creation happened out of nothing. In the early third century Hippolytus of Rome offered a clear statement of the Christian doctrine of creation.

> The one God, the first and only Deity, both Creator and Lord of all, had nothing coeval with himself, not infinite chaos, nor measureless water, nor solid earth, nor dense air, not warm fire, nor refined spirit, nor the azure canopy of the stupendous firmament. But He was One, alone in Himself. By an exercise of his will he created things that are, which antecedently had no existence, except that He willed to make them.[102]

The idea of an eternal universe would seem to have been inconsistent with the idea of Fall and Redemption which requires a linear view of history. What is important for us is that the notion of creation out of nothing implies radical freedom on the part of the Creator.

St Augustine in the fourth and fifth centuries made three attempts to complete his work on a literal reading of Genesis. Ultimately his

---
101 S.E. Baldner and W.E. Carroll (trans.), *Aquinas on Creation*, Toronto, Pontifical Institute of Medieval Studies, 1997, pp. 3-4.
102 Hippolytus, 'Refutation of All Heresies', in *Ante-Nicene Fathers*, vol. 5, eds. A. Roberts, J. Donaldson and A.C. Coxe, Buffalo, Christian Literature Co., 1886. (cf. Baldner et al, op. cit., p. 6)

commentary served as a foundation for Christian commentary on the topic. It is interesting to note that Augustine acknowledges two moments, types or instances of creation, however for the purposes of discussion of the theories of evolution, it is the original creation of the world and God's ongoing involvement in the world, with the creation of individual creatures and His intervention in the movement of the stars and the weather patterns and seasons that will be referred to here. He writes:

> ... one in the original creation when God made all creatures before resting from all his works on the seventh day, and the other in the administration of creatures by which he works even now. In the first instance God made everything together without any moments of time intervening, but now he works within the course of time, by which we see the stars move from their rising to their setting, the weather change from summer to winter ...[103]

Augustine clearly recognizes that God is continually involved in the individual creation of each being. He writes:

> For the power and light of the Creator, who rules and embraces all, makes every creature abide; and if this power ever ceased to govern creatures, their essences would pass away and all nature would perish. When the builder puts up a house and departs, his work remains in spite of the fact that he is no longer there. But the universe will pass away in the twinkling of an eye if God withdraws His ruling hand...

> We must, therefore, distinguish in the works of God those which He makes even now and those from which He rested on the seventh day. For there are some who think that only the world was made by God and that everything else is made by the world according to His ordination and

---

[103] St Augustine, *The Literal Meaning of Genesis*, op. cit., vol. 1, p. 162.

> command, but that God Himself makes nothing [other than his original act creation] ...
>
> Hence, God moves His whole creation by a hidden power, and all creatures are subject to this movement: the angels carry out His commands, the stars move in their courses, the winds blow now this way, now that, deep pools seethe with tumbling waterfalls and mists forming above them, meadows come to life as their seeds put forth the grass, animals are born and live their lives according to their proper instincts, the evil are permitted to try the just. It is thus that God unfolds the generations which He laid up in creation when first He founded it; and they would not be sent forth to run their course if He who made creatures ceased to exercise His provident rule over them.[104]

This question of God's role in the universe particularly in relation to the problem of evil led to numerous heresies, including the Manichaean heresy which was a form of Gnosticism and based on assuming that matter is fundamentally evil: the Gnostics saw the universe as a hostile place and therefore not created by an act of God. The Manichaeans held to a radical separation of the physical world from the spiritual world. They thought that the human soul belongs to God but that the human body is evil. These views were radically opposed to the Christian faith which saw God as the source of everything and all that He created as good.

The Islamic philosopher, Averroes, and the Jewish theologian and philosopher, Maimonides, were both troubled by the idea that all of creation relied upon the constant intervention of the creator. They thought that these views implicitly rejected the idea of cause and effect in nature and hence the very basis of scientific analysis. Maimonides writes:

> They assert that when a man moves a pen, it is not the man

---
[104] Ibid., pp. 171-172.

who moves it; for the motion occurring in the pen is an accident created by God in the pen. Similarly the motion of the hand, which we think of as moving the pen, is an accident created by God in the moving hand. Only, God has instead instituted the habit that the motion of the hand is commitment with the motion of the pen, without the hand exercising in any respect an influence on, or being causative in regard to, the motion of the pen.[105]

Maimonides accepts the creation out of nothing and the reliance of all creation upon God for its purpose but rejects the idea that all causation is dependent upon the direct intervention of the Creator. He writes:

> My purpose ... is to explain to you, by means of arguments that come close to being a demonstration, that what exists indicates to us of necessity that it exists in virtue of the purpose of One who purposed; and to do this without having to take upon myself what the Mutakallium have undertaken – to abolish the nature of that which exists and to adopt atomism, the opinion that according to which accidents are perpetually being created, [an opinion they adopt in order to maintain their position of divine causation] ...[106]

4.2 Doctrine on Creation of the Universe Out of Nothing

The issue of creation out of nothing was declared by the Fourth Lateran Council in 1215. The first Canon of the Council states:

> We firmly believe and openly confess that there is only one true God, eternal and immense, omnipotent, unchangeable, incomprehensible, and ineffable, Father, Son,

---

105 Maimonides, *The Guide of the Perplexed*, vol. 2, trans. S. Pines, Chicago, University of Chicago, 1963, p. 303. (cf. Baldner et al, op. cit., p. 20)
106 Ibid.

and Holy Ghost; three Persons indeed but one essence, substance, or nature absolutely simple; the Father (proceeding) from no one, but the Son from the Father only, and the Holy Ghost equally from both, always without beginning and end. The Father begetting, the Son begotten, and the Holy Ghost proceeding; consubstantial and coequal, co-omnipotent and coeternal, the one principle of the universe, Creator of all things invisible and visible, spiritual and corporeal, who from the beginning of time and by His omnipotent power made from nothing creatures both spiritual and corporeal, angelic, namely, and mundane, and then human, as it were, common, composed of spirit and body. The devil and the other demons were indeed created by God good by nature but they became bad through themselves; man, however, sinned at the suggestion of the devil. This Holy Trinity in its common essence undivided and in personal properties divided, through Moses, the holy prophets, and other servants gave to the human race at the most opportune intervals of time the doctrine of salvation.[107]

The *Catechism of the Catholic Church* sites the above text as its source for the proclamation of the creation out of nothing.[108] The Catechism also says about the universe and its creatures:

337 God himself created the visible world in all its richness, diversity and order. Scripture presents the work of the Creator symbolically as a succession of six days of divine "work", concluded by the "rest" of the seventh day. On the subject of creation, the sacred text teaches the truths revealed by God for our salvation, permitting us to "recognize the inner nature, the value and the ordering of the whole of creation to the praise of God."

---
[107] The Canons of the Fourth Lateran Council, 1215, retrieved from http://www.fordham.edu/halsall/basis/lateran4.html (accessed 18 July 2011).
[108] *Catechism of the Catholic Church*, n. 327.

338 *Nothing exists that does not owe its existence to God the Creator.* The world began when God's word drew it out of nothingness; all existent beings, all of nature, and all human history are rooted in this primordial event, the very genesis by which the world was constituted and time begun.

339 *Each creature possesses its own particular goodness and perfection.* For each one of the works of the "six days" it is said: "And God saw that it was good." "By the very nature of creation, material being is endowed with its own stability, truth and excellence, its own order and laws." Each of the various creatures, willed in its own being, reflects in its own way a ray of God's infinite wisdom and goodness. Man must therefore respect the particular goodness of every creature, to avoid any disordered use of things which would be in contempt of the Creator and would bring disastrous consequences for human beings and their environment.

340 God wills the *interdependence of creatures*. The sun and the moon, the cedar and the little flower, the eagle and the sparrow: the spectacle of their countless diversities and inequalities tells us that no creature is self-sufficient. Creatures exist only in dependence on each other, to complete each other, in the service of each other.[109]

Essential to the Christian idea of creation is that the Creator exists and is the first cause of all that exists, that creation does not involve intermediaries and that the Creator creates out of nothing. At the same time this belief in creation does not exclude the autonomy of nature and therefore the role of science in seeking to discover cause-and-effect in nature.

Compatibility between a theory of evolution and Scripture depends on making a distinction between the visible and the

---

109 Ibid.

invisible universe. Science studies the visible universe yet we can know truths about what is invisible. In *Gaudium et Spes,* Vatican II held:

> Man judges rightly that by his intellect he surpasses the material universe, for he shares in the light of the divine mind. By relentlessly employing his talents through the ages he has indeed made progress in the practical sciences and in technology and the liberal arts. In our times he has won superlative victories, especially in his probing of the material world and in subjecting it to himself. Still he has always searched for more penetrating truths, and finds them. For his intelligence is not confined to observable data alone, but can with genuine certitude attain to reality itself as knowable, though in consequence of sin that certitude is partly obscured and weakened.[110]

The challenge for those who accept the position of Pope John Paul II and Pope Benedict XVI on evolution is to find compatibility between the evidence attested to by science, about the evolution of the species, and what through faith we know of the invisible realities of our human nature and direct creation by God of our immortal souls.

4.3 St Thomas Aquinas and Creation

A matter of great interest is that St Thomas Aquinas held, as a matter of faith, the doctrine of creation out of nothing but he also believed that, as a matter of reason, God could equally have created an internal universe rather than have created it out of nothing. At the same time, however, he also thought that a universe created out of nothing still remains intelligible scientifically and that believing that the universe was created out of nothing was consistent with

---

[110] Second Vatican Council, *Gaudium et Spes*, op. cit., n. 15.

the autonomy of that creation. In this he differed from his mentor, Albert the Great. The latter held:

> It ought to be said that creation is properly a divine work. To us, moreover, it seems to be astounding in that we cannot conclude to it because it is not subject to a demonstration of reason. And so not even the philosophers have known it, unless perchance some [should have known something] from the sayings of the Prophets. But no one ever investigated it through demonstration. Some, to be sure, have found certain probable reasons, but they do not prove [creation] sufficiently.[111]

One of the earliest writings of St Thomas Aquinas is his treatment of the topic of creation in his commentary on a work of Peter Lombard, which was a popular text at the time. In his *Scriptum super libros Sententiarum magistri Petri Lombardi*, Aquinas sets out a structured analysis of the doctrine of creation beginning with the proofs of creation, the definition of creation and then how creation proceeds. All of which are directly relevant to understanding the contemporary issue of evolution in relation to creation. In order to understand whether our faith is compatible with the scientific theory of evolution we need to be clear about what, in faith, we believe.

Aquinas was much influenced by Aristotle and the latter's philosophical analysis, particularly his arguments for the view that everything that comes to be comes to be by the agency of something, from something and to be something.[112] Aristotle thought that the universe was eternal. Nonetheless Aquinas was able to use his metaphysics to argue for a first cause. If everything

---

[111] Baldner et al, op. cit. p. 27.
[112] Aristotle, *Metaphysics*, bk. VII, pt. 7, trans. W.D. Ross, retrieved from http://classics.mit.edu/Aristotle/metaphysics.7.vii.html (accessed 19 November 2011).

has a cause as Aristotle argued then there must be a first cause according to Aquinas.

4.4 The Proofs of Creation

Aquinas begins this treatment by addressing the Manichaean heresy and its difficulties with the existence of both good and evil in the world. In this view there was more than one first cause, a cause of good and a cause of evil. Aquinas argues, instead, that there can be only one truly first principle. His first argument is an argument from observation of the world around us. He argues that the motions of the heavenly bodies, in fact the entire cosmology, are according to an intelligible order in which the parts serve the purposes of each other. He argues that this could not happen unless the parts were aimed at a single goal and, therefore, that there must be one supreme final cause which is desired by all.[113]

Secondly he argues that the first principle or first cause is found in the nature of all things:

> The nature of being is found in all things, in some more nobly, in others less nobly, such that the natures of the things themselves are not the very being which they have. Otherwise, being would belong to the concept of quiddity of anything, which is false, since the quiddity of anything can be understood without understanding whether the thing exists. Natures must, therefore, have being from something else and must be ultimately a nature which is its own being, otherwise there would be an infinite regress. And this it is which gives meaning to all, and there can be only one such being, since the nature of being is of the same meaning in all according to analogy. The unity of the effect requires the unity of its essential cause.[114]

---

[113] Aquinas, *Scriptum super Libros Sententiarum Petri Lombardi*, bk. 2, dist. 1, q. 1, (cf. Baldner et al, op. cit., p. 66)
[114] Baldner et al, op. cit., pp. 66-67.

Thirdly he argues that the material world must have a material cause because there must be a summit of completeness and purity of actuality. Actuality precedes potentiality and the complete precedes the incomplete.[115] Several times in other works Aquinas returns to this topic, in *Summa Contra Gentiles* 2, in *Queastiones disputatae de potentia Dei* q. 3, and in *Summa Theologica* 1a, qq 44-46. Essentially what he has argued, in this first instance, is that there is a first cause that gives being, that is, existence, to everything in the universe.

4.5 What does "Creation" Mean?

In the second article of the work on creation, Aquinas sets out to explain what creation is, what it means to be created. There are several puzzles concerning what creation from nothing means.

First is the issue of whether creation from nothing means that a created being must have a temporal beginning; that is a beginning in time. Some, such as Anselm and Bonaventure, thought that creation excluded the possibility of an eternal being, a being with no beginning. Aquinas, however, argued that as a matter of reason it is not impossible to conceive of a being who is created but who always existed, though he concedes that as a matter of faith the universe had a temporal beginning.

Second, there is the implication of the dependence of a created being upon the Creator for its continued existence. The explanation that Aquinas gives is that the natural state of a created being is non-being because to be needs the constant causality of the Creator.

Third, there is a difference between creating out of nothing and change, such as giving form to matter. Scripture describes the creation as a creation out of nothing, not merely a change to something existing. Creation means bringing something into existence that did not previously exist.

---
115 Ibid.

Fourth, creation is relational in that there is a relationship between the creature and Creator but it is only a one-way relation. The Creator is unchangeable so the relationship is like the relationship of a knower to that which is known. The knower has no effect whatsoever on that which is known but that which is known clearly has an effect on the knower. Creation is both what the creature constantly receives from the Creator and the result of that activity.[116]

4.6 Emanation

In the third article, Aquinas addresses what is called *emanationism*, which is the notion, obviously important to theories of evolution, that a created being could emerge intermediately from another created being. That is to say whether God can use creatures as instruments in the creation of other creatures. He argues that this cannot be because an instrument is only able to cause an effect that is commensurate with its own form. In his Commentary on Sentences of Peter Lombardi, Thomas Aquinas allows for the philosophical possibility of intermediate creation, though asserting that Scripture excludes it,[117] but in the *Summa* he writes:

> It happens, however, that something participates in the proper action of another, not by its own power, but instrumentally, inasmuch as it acts by the power of another; as air can heat and ignite by the power of fire. And so some have supposed that although creation is the proper act of the universal cause, still some inferior cause acting by the power of the first cause, can create. And thus Avicenna asserted that the first separate substance created by God created another after itself, and the substance of the world and its soul; and that the substance of the world creates

---
116 Ibid.
117 Ibid.

the matter of inferior bodies. And in the same manner the Master says (Sent. iv, D, 5) that God can communicate to a creature the power of creating, so that the latter can create ministerially, not by its own power.

But such a thing cannot be, because the secondary instrumental cause does not participate in the action of the superior cause, except inasmuch as by something proper to itself it acts dispositively to the effect of the principal agent. If therefore it effects nothing, according to what is proper to itself, it is used to no purpose; nor would there be any need of certain instruments for certain actions. Thus we see that a saw, in cutting wood, which it does by the property of its own form, produces the form of a bench, which is the proper effect of the principal agent. Now the proper effect of God creating is what is presupposed to all other effects, and that is absolute being. Hence nothing else can act dispositively and instrumentally to this effect, since creation is not from anything presupposed, which can be disposed by the action of the instrumental agent. So therefore it is impossible for any creature to create, either by its own power or instrumentally – that is, ministerially.[118]

If we are to accept a theory of evolution then we must disagree with Aquinas and follow Avicenna. Clearly contemporary theories of evolution, based as they are on molecular biology and the passing on of genetic inheritance, postulate that more complex beings can evolve through mutation and the process of natural selection, that favours more complex beings for their adaptability and, hence, survivability in a competitive environment. Aquinas lacked knowledge of molecular biology and Mendellian inheritance.

---

[118] Aquinas, *Summa Theologica I*, Q. 45, Art. 5

4.7 The Stability of Creation

In article 4, Aquinas addresses what might be called the stability of creation, that is whether the continued existence of a created being requires the constant creative intervention of the Creator or whether they have, within themselves, the capacity to continue to exist. This is obviously relevant to the discussion of evolution which offers an explanation for the development of the created order from an initial beginning. At stake is the issue of whether creatures, created out of nothing, can have real causality and whether the work of the sciences in seeking to understand causality is a real science. So on the one hand, there is the faith that all created beings are dependent for their existence upon God and, on the other, there is the evidence of generation of new life and our understanding of the way in which that happens sexually, in the formation of a new genome at fertilization.

Aquinas argues that the activities of nature are dependent upon God but it is an indication of His goodness that there is autonomy of nature. This is related to our understanding of free will in which God created us the way we are, with intelligence and reason, and set us free, all the more to be in his *image and likeness* and capable in a human way of returning his love.[119] Aquinas writes in the *Summa*:

> Two things belong to providence--namely, the type of the order of things foreordained towards an end; and the execution of this order, which is called government. As regards the first of these, God has immediate providence over everything, because He has in His intellect the types of everything, even the smallest; and whatsoever causes He assigns to certain effects, He gives them the power to produce those effects. Whence it must be that He has beforehand the type of those effects in His mind. As to the

---
119 Baldner et al, op. cit. pp. 48-52.

second, there are certain intermediaries of God's providence; for He governs things inferior by superior, not on account of any defect in His power, but by reason of the abundance of His goodness; so that the dignity of causality is imparted even to creatures.[120]

And further on he writes:

... providence, of which predestination is a part, does not do away with secondary causes but so provides effects, that the order of secondary causes falls also under providence ...as natural effects are provided by God in such a way that natural causes are directed to bring about those natural effects, without which those effects would not happen ...[121]

According to Aquinas (expressing it simply), the Creator holds all things in being so that in every moment of every being there is dependence upon the Creator, but the nature of His creation is such that beings are capable of causing effects in a way that are Divinely ordained.

4.8 Eternal or Temporal Being

In article 5, Aquinas returns to the topic discussed in article 2 in relation to whether, as a matter of philosophical reasoning, we can determine whether the universe was always eternal or whether it had a temporal beginning. Aquinas addresses the argument that it necessarily is eternal and the alternative argument that it necessarily has a temporal beginning. He argues that either is possible and the fact that the universe has been created does not, in itself, make it necessary for it to be eternal nor to have a temporal beginning. He concludes that having a temporal beginning is not

---
120 Aquinas, *Summa Theologica I*, Q. 22, Art. 3.
121 Ibid., Q. 23, Art. 8.

necessary but is simply a matter of faith based on revelation.[122] This is most interesting for understanding the complementary roles of faith and reason, especially our task of evangelization as Christians.

4.9 An Exegesis of Genesis

In article 6, having addressed the philosophical and theological arguments about the nature of creation, Aquinas then sets out to do an exegesis on the Genesis account of creation. A problem with understanding the Genesis 1 account is that the phrase "In the beginning ..." can have several different meanings.

First, it would refer to the first principle or first cause, which, in the light of John's Gospel, would be a reference to Christ as the second person of the Trinity. Thus in the Genesis 1 account "In the beginning ..." is directly linked to John's account, "In the beginning there was the Word ..."[123]

Second, "In the beginning ..." may simply refer to the first moment. That is the beginning of time.

Third, "In the beginning ..." may refer not to the first moment but that period of time before things were created.

Aquinas uses each of these meanings to address a particular heresy. The first, about the first cause, addresses the Manichaean heresy of there being multiple causes, the good and the evil. The second addresses the heresy that the universe is necessarily eternal and so had no beginning. And the third addresses the heresy that visible things were created through the mediation of spiritual creatures.[124] In other words he engages all three meanings of the phrase, "In the beginning ...".

---

122 Ibid.
123 Baldner et al, op. cit., pp. 106-107 (footnote).
124 Ibid., p. 108.

4.10 Compatibility with Scripture

Evolutionary theory holds that the species evolved from some beginning. The Big Bang theory is offered as an explanation of that beginning, though the Big Bang theory and evolutionary theory are two distinct theories and evolutionary theory is not dependent upon the Big Bang theory. The evolution of the cosmos and the evolution of species are different matters. The theory of natural selection applies only to life forms, forms that reproduce and die.

The story of creation, told to us in Scripture, is essentially an account of our origin; our having been created in the beginning by God. According to Aquinas, an understanding of creation is consistent with an understanding of cause and effect that is central to the work of the human sciences.

Whether the world began with an uncaused Big Bang or whether it began by an act of creation, as the cause of that beginning, is not able to be determined by science. Somehow, the idea of a Creator seems more intelligible than what seem to be the alternatives to a Creator, something happening out of nothing of its own accord or the idea of eternal matter somehow acquiring form. Aquinas argues philosophically for the view that there must be a Creator. What is clear, whether or not you accept the philosophical argument for a first cause, is that science is unable to determine the origin of the universe and that claims about evolutionary theory having established the fact that there is no Creator are not scientific claims.

According to the account that Aquinas has given of creation, our faith in creation is consistent with a scientific theory of evolution; though, of course, Aquinas did not ever address the issue of evolutionary theory as it is currently understood. However, there are questions for faith in our seeking to achieve compatibility between faith and a theory of evolution.

As discussed in Chapter 2, one of the issues, obviously, is

whether the evolution of man applies only to man's body, as seems to be the position adopted by the Vatican Council I and by Popes Benedict XVI and John Paul II. (The Second Vatican Council did not seem to address the issue.) If the soul is a result of a direct creative intervention by God then that creates some difficulties for the doctrine proclaimed at the Council of Vienne, that the soul is the form of the body and informs the matter that is the body. It is not impossible that God intervenes at the point of each conception, when the child begins, and immediately creates an immortal soul. It is also conceivable that at the point that an animal gave birth to a mutant and that mutant was a human being then God chose that moment to create a human soul for the first time.

The problem, however, is that the doctrine proclaimed at the Council of Vienne holds that the human immortal soul does more than just provide the faculty of reason: it is that which informs and forms the matter that is the human body. So we have an account of matter developing, through mutation and natural selection, a form that determines the inherited features of each creature, including human beings, yet at that point a human soul is created which makes us *imago Dei*. We are in need of an account to explain the transition from an animal soul, developed by evolution, to a human soul individually created at conception, when the first new genome of the new human being is formed. There is seemingly a gap in our understanding and a wonderful topic for a PhD to attempt to fill!

A second issue concerns our understanding of the Fall and the belief that death and other aspects of our fallen state are the consequence of sin. The puzzle is that in evolutionary theory death is very much part of the evolution of the species before man arrives on the scene and introduces sin to the world.

In relation to the first issue, the *Catechism of the Catholic Church* teaches:

> **365** The unity of soul and body is so profound that one has to consider the soul to be the "form" of the body: i.e., it is because of its spiritual soul that the body made of matter becomes a living, human body; spirit and matter, in man, are not two natures united, but rather their union forms a single nature.
>
> **366** The Church teaches that every spiritual soul is created immediately by God – it is not "produced" by the parents – and also that it is immortal: it does not perish when it separates from the body at death, and it will be reunited with the body at the final Resurrection.

The source given for the former is the Council of Vienne and for the latter the encyclical by Pius XII *Humani Generis*, Paul VI *Credo of the People of God* n. 8 and the Fifth Lateran Council. These therefore are confirmed doctrines of the Church.

Pope Paul VI writes in *Solemni Hac Liturgia,* known also as the *"Credo of the People of God"*:

> 8. We believe in one only God, Father, Son and Holy Spirit, creator of things visible such as this world in which our transient life passes, of things invisible such as the pure spirits which are also called angels, and creator in each man of his spiritual and immortal soul.

4.11 Death and the Fall

The issue of death following the Fall has its basis in the passage, Genesis 2:15-17:

> The LORD God took the man and put him in the Garden of Eden to work it and take care of it. And the LORD God commanded the man, "You are free to eat from any tree in the garden; but you must not eat from the tree of the knowledge of good and evil, for when you eat from it you will certainly die."

In the Beginning ...

The puzzle is that the theory of evolution is based on competition for survival, so there was death before man evolved and hence before there could be sin. One way of handling this is to refer to the death caused by sin as spiritual death as many theologians have chosen to do: the death of having turned away from God.

The *Catechism*, citing *Gaudium et Spes* n. 13 as the authority, claims that the Fall affirms a primeval event, a deed that took place "at the beginning of the history of man",[125] and that Revelation gives us the certainty of faith that the whole of human history is marked by the original fault freely committed by our first parents. However *Gaudium et Spes* is not so categorical. It states:

> Although he was made by God in a state of holiness, from the very onset of his history man abused his liberty, at the urging of the Evil One. Man set himself against God and sought to attain his goal apart from God. Although they knew God, they did not glorify Him as God, but their senseless minds were darkened and they served the creature rather than the Creator. [Rom 1:21-5] What divine revelation makes known to us agrees with experience. Examining his heart, man finds that he has inclinations toward evil too, and is engulfed by manifold ills which cannot come from his good Creator. Often refusing to acknowledge God as his beginning, man has disrupted also his proper relationship to his own ultimate goal as well as his whole relationship toward himself and others and all created things.[126]

This reading is consistent with St Paul's letter to the *Romans* 1:18-25 where he writes:

> The wrath of God is being revealed from heaven against all the godlessness and wickedness of people, who

---

[125] *Catechism of the Catholic Church*, n. 390.
[126] Second Vatican Council, *Gaudium et Spes*, op. cit., n. 13.

suppress the truth by their wickedness, since what may be known about God is plain to them, because God has made it plain to them. For since the creation of the world God's invisible qualities – his eternal power and divine nature – have been clearly seen, being understood from what has been made, so that people are without excuse.

For although they knew God, they neither glorified him as God nor gave thanks to him, but their thinking became futile and their foolish hearts were darkened. Although they claimed to be wise, they became fools and exchanged the glory of the immortal God for images made to look like a mortal human being and birds and animals and reptiles.

Therefore God gave them over in the sinful desires of their hearts to sexual impurity for the degrading of their bodies with one another. They exchanged the truth about God for a lie, and worshipped and served created things rather than the Creator – who is forever praised. Amen.

In *Romans* 5:12-13 St Paul claims that death entered the world through sin.

Therefore, just as sin entered the world through one man, and death through sin, and in this way death came to all people, because all sinned –

To be sure, sin was in the world before the law was given, but sin is not charged against anyone's account where there is no law. Nevertheless, death reigned from the time of Adam to the time of Moses, even over those who did not sin by breaking a command, as did Adam, who is a pattern of the one to come.

This would seem to indicate that the death consequence is a result of sin. The idea that this means spiritual death rather than physical death seems to give more sense to the Genesis passage because when Adam and Eve did eat the fruit they did not immediately die, but they did suffer the consequences of sin.

In *1 Corinthians* 15: 20-22, St Paul writes: "But Christ has indeed been raised from the dead, the first fruits of those who have fallen asleep. For since death came through a man, the resurrection of the dead comes also through a man. For as in Adam all die, so in Christ all will be made alive."

However it is argued that the passage is more meaningful if spiritual death is meant rather than physical death. Also, as in Romans 5, here the term death refers to *human* death rather than animal death, as there is no indication that animals are resurrected.

In Ephesians chapter 2:1-5, St Paul writes:

> As for you, you were dead in your transgressions and sins, in which you used to live when you followed the ways of this world and of the ruler of the kingdom of the air, the spirit who is now at work in those who are disobedient. All of us also lived among them at one time, gratifying the cravings of our flesh and following its desires and thoughts. Like the rest, we were by nature deserving of wrath. But because of his great love for us, God, who is rich in mercy, made us alive with Christ even when we were dead in transgressions – it is by grace you have been saved.

This would seem to indicate that the death of original sin was a spiritual death, a state of fearful depravation from which we are rescued by Jesus, thus making "death" of original sin figurative rather than actual. Likewise in Romans 8:6, Paul writes that to be carnally-minded is death but to be spiritually-minded is life and peace.

On the other hand, the Second Vatican Council seems to be explicit about real bodily death being due to the Fall:

In addition, that bodily death from which man would have been immune had he not sinned will be vanquished, according to the Christian faith, when man who was ruined by his own doing is restored to wholeness by an almighty and merciful Saviour. For God has called man and still calls him so that with his entire being he might be joined to Him in an endless sharing of a divine life beyond all corruption. Christ won this victory when He rose to life, for by His death He freed man from death.[127]

St Augustine wrote that death and concupiscence are the result of original sin.

> This death occurred on the day when our first parents did what God had forbidden. Their bodies lost the privileged condition they had had, a condition mysteriously maintained by nourishment from the tree of life, which would have been able to preserve them from sickness and from the aging process. For although they had natural bodies which were to be transformed subsequently, yet even there in Paradise, in the food from the tree of life, there was a symbol of what happens through the spiritual nourishment given by Wisdom ...
>
> When Adam and Eve, therefore, lost their privileged state, their bodies became subject to disease and death, like the bodies of animals, and consequently subject to the same drive by which there is in animals a desire to copulate and thus provide for offspring to take the place of those that die. Nevertheless, even in its punishment the rational soul gave evidence of its innate nobility when it blushed because of the animal movement of the members of its body and when it imparted to it a sense of shame, not only because it began to experience something where there had been no such feeling before, but also because

---

[127] Second Vatican Council, *Gaudium et Spes*, op. cit., n. 18.

this movement of which it was ashamed came from the violation of the divine command.[128]

Pope John Paul II also seems to read the death from the Fall as real death. He writes:

> The horizon of death extends over the whole perspective of human life on earth, life that was inserted in that original biblical cycle of "knowledge-generation." Man has broken the covenant with his Creator by picking the fruit of the tree of the knowledge of good and evil. He is detached by God-Yahweh from the tree of life: "Now, let him not put forth his hand and take also of the tree of life, and eat, and live forever" (Gen 3:21). In this way, the life given to man in the mystery of creation has not been taken away. But it is restricted by the limit of conceptions, births and deaths, and further aggravated by the perspective of hereditary sinfulness. But it is given to him again, in a way, as a task in the same ever-recurring cycle.[129]

I am not sure how the Genesis passage should be read. However if it means real death then this creates a difficulty for compatibility, unless the death of animals and the death of humans are separated, so that only animals died before the Fall and a consequence of the Fall was that man became like the animals.

I offer these questions for thought because there is much work to be done to explore compatibility between the Scriptural understanding of creation and a theory of evolution. There are significant explanations needed if we are to account for compatibility between faith and science in relation to our origins, including not just the evolution of the human biological species from animals but also the ordinary human reproduction of offspring

---

[128] St Augustine, *The Literal Meaning of Genesis*, chapter 32.
[129] Pope John Paul II, 'Theology of the Body' Catechesis, *L'Osservatore Romano*, 31 Mar 1980.

from human parents and the nature of the dynamic unity between body and soul that is the human person. There is so much also to be understood about the effects of sin and redemption. There is so much work to be done, and that is very exciting!

5

INTRINSIC AND INSTRUMENTAL VALUE AND ANTHROPOCENTRISM

5.1 Intrinsic and Instrumental Good

When we say that something is good we are commending it. We may do so because it is good *for* something or because it is simply good, good in itself. We might, for instance, say "This is a good knife". What we would mean is that the knife has properties that make it useful for doing the things for which we use a knife; that is to say, we might be praising it because it is sharp, or that it holds its edge, or that it is a useful size for a particular task, or it has a strong blade such as needed for cutting raw pumpkin, or a sharp flexible blade such as needed for boning chicken. Good in that case means good for something, or *instrumentally* good.

However, if we are commenting on a painting and saying that it is good, it is more likely to be a statement meaning that it is good in itself; that it is *intrinsically* good. Such a statement would reflect an aesthetic judgment. "Good" however could also be a moral judgment. The philosopher, William Frankena, provided a list of things that he thought were valuable in themselves, that is to say, they were *intrinsically* valuable. The list included: life, consciousness, and activity; health and strength; pleasures and satisfactions of all or certain kinds; happiness, beatitude, contentment, etc.; truth; knowledge and true opinions of various kinds, understanding, wisdom; beauty, harmony, proportion in objects contemplated; aesthetic experience; morally good dispositions or virtues; mutual affection, love, friendship, cooperation; just distribution of goods and evils; harmony and proportion in one's own life; power and experiences of achievement; self-expression; freedom; peace, security; adventure and novelty; and good reputation, honor and esteem.[130]

Some have tried to capture the distinction between something being intrinsically good and something being instrumentally good by reference to ends and means. Something is instrumentally good because it is a means to something else. Something is intrinsically good when it is an end in itself.[131]

Frankena puzzled over whether intrinsic goodness pertained only to the *experience* of something that is good, or whether goodness had properties of its own independent of its being experienced. Is a forest beautiful in itself or is its beauty only in the way in which it is perceived? There'll be more about this later when we talk about "Beauty and Creation".

Other puzzles concern whether intrinsic goods are transitive. That is to say if A is intrinsically better than something else B, which is itself intrinsically better than some third thing C, cannot it be that A is not intrinsically better than C? In other words is intrinsic goodness a property that can be compared or are we talking about quite different things when we compare different intrinsic goods. Is there a hierarchy of goods such that some are considered better than others or are they incommensurate?[132]

G.E. Moore claimed that there is a principle of organic unity such that the intrinsic value of a whole must not be assumed to be

---

130 William K. Frankena, *Ethics*, 2nd ed., Englewood Cliffs, Prentice Hall 1973, chapter 5, retrieved from http://www.ditext.com/frankena/e5.html (accessed 2010-2014).
131 Ibid.
132 'Intrinsic vs. Extrinsic Value', *The Stanford Encyclopaedia of Philosophy*, 2010, http://plato.stanford.edu/archives/win2010/entries/value-intrinsic-extrinsic, (accessed 2010-2014).

the same as the sum of the intrinsic values of its parts.[133] An object may be considered beautiful even though its parts may not. The goodness may be in the organic whole, in the coming together of the parts. The single note of a trumpet might not be considered beautiful but becomes vitally so within a concerto.

5.2 The Environment and Anthropocentrism

Debate over environmental ethics has often focused on the issue of whether the environment is intrinsically or instrumentally valuable. Those who hold that it is only instrumentally valuable are considered to adopt an anthropocentric view, the view that the environment is only valuable insofar as it serves human purposes. This view seems to be reflected in the Vatican II document *Gaudium et Spes* when the Council writes:

> God intended the earth with everything contained in it for the use of all human beings and peoples. Thus, under the leadership of justice and in the company of charity, created goods should be in abundance for all in like manner. Whatever the forms of property may be, as adapted to the legitimate institutions of peoples, according to diverse and changeable circumstances, attention must always be paid to this universal destination of earthly goods. In using them, therefore, man should regard the external things that he legitimately possesses not only as his own but also as common in the sense that they should be able to benefit not only him but also others. On the other hand, the right of having a share of earthly goods sufficient for oneself and one's family belongs to everyone.[134]

On the other hand, Pope John Paul II takes his cue on this

---

[133] P.A. Schilpp (ed.), *The Philosophy of G.E. Moore*, Evanston, Northwestern University Press, 1942.
[134] Second Vatican Council, *Guadium et Spes*, op. cit., n. 69.

issue from the Genesis account of Creation and the recurring refrain, *"... and God saw that it was good"*, repeated after God creates each element of the universe. After the creation of man and woman the holy writer says, *"... and God saw that it was very good"* (Gen 1:31).

On the Pope's interpretation of the Genesis story he refers to humanity having been given dominion over creation but disturbing its order through sin. Thus he writes:

> Christians believe that the Death and Resurrection of Christ accomplished the work of reconciling humanity to the Father, who "was pleased ... through (Christ) to reconcile to himself *all things*, whether on earth or in heaven, making peace by the blood of his cross" (*Col* 1:19-20). Creation was thus made new (cf. *Rev* 21:5). Once subjected to the bondage of sin and decay (cf. *Rom* 8:21), it has now received new life while "we wait for new heavens and a new earth in which righteousness dwells" (2 *Pt* 3:13). Thus, the Father "has made known to us in all wisdom and insight the mystery ... which he set forth in Christ as a plan for the fullness of time, to unite *all things* in him, all things in heaven and things on earth" (*Eph* 1:9-10).[135]

Thus John Paul II spoke of the need for us to seek peace with all creation by respecting the order that God gave to it:

> When man turns his back on the Creator's plan, he provokes a disorder which has inevitable repercussions on the rest of the created order. If man is not at peace with God, then earth itself cannot be at peace: "Therefore the land mourns and all who dwell in it languish, and also the

---

135 Pope John Paul II, Message for the World Day of Peace, *Peace with God the Creator, Peace with All Creation*, 1990, n. 5, http://www.vatican.va/holy_father/john_paul_ii/messages/peace/documents/hf_jp-ii_mes_19891208_xxiii-world-day-for-peace_en.html (accessed 2010-2014).

beasts of the field and the birds of the air and even the fish of the sea are taken away" (*Hos* 4:3).[136]

In his encyclical *Caritas in Veritate*, Pope Benedict XVI writes similarly about the importance of respecting the order and design that God has given to all creation:

> Today the subject of development is also closely related to the duties arising from *our relationship to the natural environment*. The environment is God's gift to everyone, and in our use of it we have a responsibility towards the poor, towards future generations and towards humanity as a whole. When nature, including the human being, is viewed as the result of mere chance or evolutionary determinism, our sense of responsibility wanes. In nature, the believer recognizes the wonderful result of God's creative activity, which we may use responsibly to satisfy our legitimate needs, material or otherwise, while respecting the intrinsic balance of creation. If this vision is lost, we end up either considering nature an untouchable taboo or, on the contrary, abusing it. Neither attitude is consonant with the Christian vision of nature as the fruit of God's creation.[137]

The Pope writes that in nature God has expressed his *design of love and truth*. The natural universe was given to us to be the setting for our life and it speaks to us of the Creator (cf. Rom 1:20) and his love for humanity.

In Ephesians (1:9-10), St Paul has it that God made known to us the mystery of His will according to His good pleasure, which He purposed in Christ, to be put into effect when the times reach their fulfilment – to bring unity to all things in heaven and on

---

[136] Ibid.
[137] Pope Benedict XVI, *Caritas in Veritate*, 29 June 2009, n. 48, http://www.vatican.va/holy_father/benedict_xvi/encyclicals/documents/hf_ben-xvi_enc_20090629_caritas-in-veritate_en.html (accessed 2010-2014).

earth under Christ. In Colossians (1:19-20), St Paul teaches: "For God was pleased to have all his fullness dwell in him, and through him to reconcile to himself all things, whether things on earth or things in heaven, by making peace through his blood, shed on the cross."

Pope Benedict interprets these passages as meaning that all of the universe will be "recapitulated in Christ" at the end of time. The phrase seems to have an origin in St Irenaeus who refers to Christ recapitulating Adam but at every point correcting his mistakes:

> ... when he was incarnate and became a human being he recapitulated in himself (*in seipso recapitulavit*) the long history of the human race, obtaining salvation for us that we might regain in Jesus Christ what we had lost in Adam, that is being made in the image and likeness of God.[138]

However Pope Benedict XVI writes not just of Adam in this way, but all creation:

> *Nature expresses a design of love and truth.* It is prior to us, and it has been given to us by God as the setting for our life. Nature speaks to us of the Creator (cf. Rom 1:20) and his love for humanity. It is destined to be "recapitulated" in Christ at the end of time (cf. Eph 1:9-10; Col 1:19-20). Thus it too is a "vocation". Nature is at our disposal not as "a heap of scattered refuse", but as a gift of the Creator who has given it an inbuilt order, enabling man to draw from it the principles needed in order "to till it and keep it" (Gen 2:15).[139]

How we understand this depends on how we understand the Fall. The latter would seem, at least, to mean disunity, disharmony and confusion in relation to nature. This fits with our more modern

---

138 Alistair E. McGrath (ed.), *The Christian Theology Reader*, 3rd ed., Blackwell 2007, p. 344.
139 Pope Benedict XVI, *Caritas in Veritate*, op. cit., n. 48.

consciousness of sustainability and the non-renewable effects of some of the things that we have done to creation. Just as in being redeemed by Christ we pursue communion with God now in this life so we should pursue unity and harmony with all creation in this life. Creation suffers from our sins and in seeking unity with God we should seek unity with His Creation.

This is the theme of Pope John Paul's *Peace with God the Creator, Peace with All Creation* and of his teaching that Christ came not just to redeem mankind but to redeem all creation. He wrote that the commitment of believers to keep a healthy environment for everyone stems directly from their belief in God the Creator, from their recognition of the effects of original and personal sin, and from the certainty of having been redeemed by Christ. Respect for life and for the dignity of the human person extends also to the rest of creation, which is called to join man in praising God (cf. *Ps* 148:96).[140]

5.3 Dominion and Stewardship

Thus, in our dominion or stewardship of the earth, which includes its creatures, we are called to respect it for its own sake and not to exploit it as simply something given to us for our own purposes. We should value it not just because it would be better for us if we managed it well, but because it too is created by God, it is good and, like us, reflects His divine nature.

This is not to say that the needs of the environment are more important than human beings. As rational creatures we are the pinnacle of God's creation. According to Genesis, in making us God declared us to be "very good"; we are told that we are made in His image and likeness. However, we are also called to respect all of God's creation; our stewardship requires us to try to understand

---

140 Pope John Paul II, *Peace with God the Creator, Peace with All Creation*, op. cit., n. 16.

His design and purpose for every creature and to act in accord with that design and purpose.

This makes the science of ecology a vital science, not just because we depend on the environment but because it too is intrinsically good. Science seeks to understand something that is good not merely useful.

On this view of stewardship, anthropocentrism is a mistake. In God's plan, the universe does not exist merely for us but with us; we need to learn to live in balance with it and its needs if we are to be at peace. The exploitation of the environment in unsustainable ways is not just foolhardy, in relation to the needs of future generations, it is a failure to respect God's will. Exploitation is based on treating the environment as merely good instrumentally rather than intrinsically.

Obviously, the issue of evolution and creation is of great relevance to the way in which we see the universe and whether we see it as intrinsically valuable or merely instrumentally valuable; because the world was created by God and retains within it His design and purpose, there is no permit for us to treat it merely instrumentally but to treat it according to the design and purpose that God has meant for it. In this discussion of creation and evolution, it has been shown that evolutionary theory does not exclude the possibility that God designed and intended the universe to develop the way that it has. It is the case that some who support the theory of evolution also claim that the universe developed as a result of chance and natural selection and that the process excludes the possibility of the world and the universe being a result of God's design. However, such a view is not a scientific view but an ideological one and not at all supported by the evidence.

On the other hand, those who treat the Genesis account as literal also hold that the theory of evolution excludes the possibility of God as Creator because on their account the universe was created in six days and was instantly created, rather than that life developed from nonlife and that the species evolved one from another until human life developed. In this discussion of evolution, it was explained that the importance of the Scriptural account is in insisting that the universe and humanity within it are created by God according to His design and purpose. In a sense, this important meaning runs parallel to the scientific theory of evolution, neither affirmed nor negated by it. We can accept, on the one hand, that God created the universe according to his design and purpose and, also, that the evidence which supports the theory of evolution is consistent with that of creation. In other words, God created matter and the laws by which it would evolve into life and eventually into human life.

Accepting this account of evolution poses no more difficulty for the individual creation of each human soul by God than does ordinary human reproduction, in which life is generated as a result of intimacy between spouses and even between those who are not married. Sometimes God even creates new life as a consequence of rape. So in the biological events of ordinary reproduction new life is generated. Christians accept this biology, alongside the theology and the belief that God supports and sustains all creation, creates each individual life and gives it an immortal soul. There would seem to be no problem in extending that biological understanding to include the possibility of human bodily life evolving from animal life and life itself evolving from nonlife. That there is a divine design and plan in the way in which evolution has developed is not excluded by the biological account though, of course, biological science has no evidence for divine intervention or, even, that there exists a human soul for each human individual. At the same time biological science has no evidence to disprove the involvement of the Creator in the evolution of the universe or to disprove the existence of a human soul. They are in effect parallel worlds, so to speak, the world of theology and the world of natural science. As the Congregation for the Doctrine of the Faith expressed it:

> Right from fertilization is begun the adventure of a human life, and each of its great capacities requires time ... to find its place and to be in a position to act. This teaching remains valid and is further confirmed, if confirmation were needed, by recent findings of human biological science which recognize that in the zygote resulting from fertilization the biological identity of a new human individual is already constituted. Certainly no experimental datum can be in itself sufficient to bring us to the recognition of a spiritual soul; nevertheless, the conclusions of science regarding the human embryo provide a valuable indication for discerning by the use of reason a personal presence at the moment of this first appearance of a human life: how could a human individual not be a human person? The Magisterium has not expressly committed itself to an affirmation of a philosophical nature, but it constantly reaffirms the moral condemnation of any kind of procured abortion. This teaching has not been changed and is unchangeable.[141]

There are thus two aspects of our created universe, the visible and the invisible. Science explores the visible aspects of the universe and theology is concerned about the invisible. The visible can be measured and tested but the invisible is beyond scientific analysis.

When we observe the great beauty, complexity and intricacy of the universe around us, and of ourselves, we can see both God's design and the results of a process over millions of years, in which the circumstances have been favourable for the molecules of life to have been formed, reproduced and developed by this

---
141 Congregation for the Doctrine of the Faith, *Donum Vitae*, op. cit.

process which has tended towards greater complexity through the effects of natural selection. A scientist may choose to see this either as a process of chance or as a process following natural laws established by God; neither explanation is provable by the evidence. Belief in God is a matter of faith and the important aspect of that faith is belief in a God who loves us and loves all His creation. Evolutionary theory is not based on a series of chance happenings resulting in growing complexity until a human being evolves. Rather evolution depends on random change that is, then, directed by the laws of natural selection that favour complexity; and where complexity provides a survival advantage. That man would evolve was not a matter of chance but a consequence of the natural laws that favoured the survival of change which was more complex and which was selected for its capacity for survival advantage. Also it remains an open question as to whether all that we experience can be accounted for by the process of natural selection. When we see a beautiful sunset or a mountain range, we have the capacity to appreciate its beauty and it appears to us to be beautiful. It is difficult to explain how our being selected for survival yielded such a capacity or how the cosmos could be so beautiful. When we experience human reason, what we experience goes well beyond the capacities needed for survival. Our intelligence includes capacities that have no connection with survival needs. Natural selection leaves much unexplained. This is not to say that reason and aesthetic experience cannot be explained as natural phenomena, only that natural selection does not explain their origins.

5.4 Is a Creator Logically Necessary?

As discussed earlier, St Thomas Aquinas offers several proofs for the existence of God including what is often called the cosmological argument. The cosmological argument is that there has to be a First

Cause. Aquinas, following Aristotle, draws a distinction between contingent existence and necessary existence. Something has necessary existence if it exists in all possible worlds.

Aquinas argues for the proposition that there has to be a first cause by supposing the contrary, that all things are contingent; that is to say, to suppose that all things can go out of existence. If this is so then there must be a time when all things go out of existence. If this was a real possibility then it would have happened and there would be nothing; but had that happened it would follow that nothing now exists. The fact that this is not so means that something exists necessarily. Our sense perceptions and experience tell us that something exists, something is there and therefore everything has not ever gone out of existence. So, all things cannot be contingent.

Aquinas also argues that everything that happens must have a cause, what he calls the principle of sufficient reason. That is to say, nothing happens without something causing it to happen. On that basis there must have been a first cause or there would be nothing. For Aquinas, this explanation leads to an assertion about there being a first cause and he suggests that that first cause is God, the self-explaining necessary existence upon which all things are contingent in all possible worlds.[142]

That there is a first cause is consistent with the theory of evolution. Consistent with a first cause is the argument that God, as that first cause, initiates the universe and the laws by which it is governed and, from that point, matter is formed with the capacity over millions of years to generate life and that life has the capacity over further millions of years to generate human life.

What biological science cannot do is identify that first cause. There is also uncertainty about the development of each individual

---

142 Pagewise Inc., *The Cosmological Argument of Aquinas*, http://www.essortment.com/all/aquinascosmolog_rend.htm (accessed 2010-2014).

species. We know that the mechanisms of both mutation and population drift can cause changes to species and the development of new species and that the process of natural selection will make those mutations survive only if they are fit to survive. That is to say natural selection is a process which selects for greater fitness and for greater complexity because greater functions give a species greater capacity to adapt to an environment and to changes in the environment.

It is interesting that the language of biology tends to ascribe purposes to the various functions that species have, even though the biological account would imply that there are no purposes but just a selection process and chance happenings through mutation. However, seeing a purpose for each of the species in the universe and understanding them as living in an ecological balance is biologically sound; this leaves open the possibility that this design and purpose may be a result of intentional planning by the Creator who first established the matter of the universe and the laws that would govern its development.

Darwin suggested that we imagine a perfectly constructed golf course in which the only variable, in determining whether the ball sank into the hole that was constructed for it, was the way in which you struck the ball. If your striking of the ball was unintelligent, uninformed and, therefore, random then you might never, in fact, sink the ball. On the other hand, if the course designers so shape the course that the green slopes towards the hole then it becomes much more likely that you will sink the ball if the game goes on for long enough. Natural selection consists of a process like the slope that directs the process towards greater complexity. Evolution relies on chance but not entirely; the rules are weighted toward advancing complexity through greater survival chances. An issue is whether those rules are also the result of chance or whether they are planned.

For us in seeing design and purpose of the Creator in the entire universe, a crucial issue, then, is how we should see each of the species and the universe itself. In admiring the complexity, the intricacy and the beauty of God's creation we see the greatness of what He has achieved; all the more so because all this developed from simple matter in the first instance. In believing in a first cause, a divine Creator, we have also the history of His relationship with humanity given to us by the holy writers in Scripture. Of course, as an historical account there are gaps and, in studying Scripture, we try to seek consistency for the explanation of that relationship but not, of course, to seek an exact chronology of human events; we read it as a complete story that includes Jesus, who alone provides meaning for the purpose of creation.

The biological sciences are thus very important for showing us the design and purpose that underlies what we have come to know as ecological balance. Everything relates to everything else and it is important for us to understand those relationships in order not to disrupt this wonderful complexity that God has given us. We stand at the pinnacle of God's creation having emerged through a process, which over millions of years, has developed greater and greater complexity, until we came to being human and to actually reflecting the image and likeness of God through our capacity to reason. We have, within our own power, capacities to preserve or to disrupt the systems that surround us in our universe.

Our understanding of God's creation which surrounds us and our capacity to exercise dominion or stewardship is crucial to ecological awareness and the development of an environmental ethic. It is important, in seeing the universe as the fruit of God's creation, that we recognize the intrinsic worth of our ecological systems and the trust that God has placed in us to protect and to safeguard His creation.

It is truly wonderful to reflect upon the identity, the role and the place of humanity within creation and the fact that, because we have reason, we can affect the evolutionary process from this point on and the nature of the universe that we and future generations will inhabit. The process of evolution goes on with us taking a part but, because we are rational, we are not the unwitting subjects of processes that are beyond our control.

5.5 The Strength of our Stewardship

It is extraordinary to think, that in giving us rationality, God has placed us in this position of being able to interfere with the balance and the laws of nature that are of His design. When we become parents, we have the power to be co-creators with God; but there is another sense in which we are co-creators with God because by what we do, the way we use energy and resources, the way in which we treat the great forests and oceans of the world and the mineral and fauna resources, we can affect what the future development of this universe, or at least this part of this universe, will be.

By seeing the universe as God's creation and its development according to the laws of nature which He designed and by understanding our own place within that creation we are able either to work with God's design or to disrupt it; we thus cease to treat the environment as merely existing for our own use. The environment and the balance of the ecologies within it are intrinsically valuable because they reflect God's design. We are not the passive recipients of God's munificence. Rather, we can seek to understand and to work with His design or we can treat the environment instrumentally to serve only our own purposes, and, in that way, risk intervening in ways that may be destructive and not in accord with that design.

Much of the risk to the environment is on a large scale such as the effects of production of energy, mining, manufacturing, management of the rivers, commercial fishing, transport and agriculture. One of the problems of the climate change debate is not only the difficulty of discerning the truth from the competing scientific claims but also of identifying how each of us could make a significant difference. Apart from who we vote for, the discretion we have seems to be in relation to the product choices and the purchases we make relative to the environmental impact of manufacturing and transport of the different choices.

5.6 Teleology

Underlying debate about environmental ethics is a notion of teleology; the idea that the universe, the creatures within it, down to the smallest least significant life form, or element of a life form, have a role and purpose. Evolutionary theory understands that different creatures have different roles within a balanced ecological system. There is a food chain and complex relationships that serve to preserve it. The excreta of one life form feeds another and that life feeds another until the circle is complete, with the first excreting animal feeding the creatures that were necessary for the development of its food source. The water that falls as rain is used by plants and animals for growth before being released to flow into the rivers, lakes and seas to evaporate or to be respired by animals directly and so be taken into the atmosphere to fall again as rain. Another example is of carbon dioxide being produced by animals, then being absorbed by plants and then released as oxygen into the atmosphere, with the carbon product being eaten as plant material by those animals which are forming another cyclic chain to keep the ecology in balance.

There is teleology for each element in the ecology. It has a function or several functions that make its existence important for the whole. Darwin's theory of evolution, that offered an explanation based on chance mutation and the laws of evolution, were thought by some to explain away the need for an overall design by a creator for ecological balance and for the purpose that each part played in achieving it. There are several different views in this respect:

- Teleomentalism is the view that recognizing or ascribing purposes to natural phenomena within the ecology is simply mental shorthand and unnecessary. We could equally explain the relationships without implying a overall design by a creator.
- Teleonaturalism is the view that purpose or meaning exists but only in a biological sense that can be explained by biological happenstance rather than by design.
- Natural Selection Analyses of Function is a view that has three separate components:
  1. Functional claims in biology are intended to explain the existence or maintenance of a trait in a given population;
  2. Biological functions are causally relevant to the existence or maintenance of traits via the mechanism of natural selection;
  3. Functional claims in biology are fully grounded in natural selection and are not derivative of psychological uses of notions such as design, intention, and purpose.
- Function and Design are used in a circular fashion in which a trait is naturally designed for X if and only if X is a biological function of that trait. Design is thus expressed as a consequence of being a biological function.
- Adaptation, Exaptation and Co-opted Use are three quite different concepts to apply to a function. If a function

evolves to provide an advantage then it indicates that the species has adapted to the environment through advantageous change, as distinct from exaptation which is a function that happens through mutation but is not necessarily an advantage. A co-opted function refers to a change that has happened and is then put to advantage by the creature and hence is an improvement but that improvement is unrelated to survival and the change is thus not due to natural selection.[143]

Underlying this discussion is the notion of teleology or purpose and whether evolution is by chance or by design according to rules that have been planned.

Whether or not there is a design by which human beings have evolved does not seem to be something that can be concluded as a matter of evidence; neither, it seems, can this be concluded as a matter of faith. For Christians, our faith in a Creator holds that it is by design.

If we and all creation exist in the way that we do according to a design, then each creature and each part of each creature has a purpose or purposes. Each exists for a reason or reasons. This makes a significant difference to the way in which we treat all of creation. In having a divine teleology, each has a place which we should respect. Utilizing a creature for reasons not consistent with the divine teleology would be problematic. Thus each creature has an intrinsic value related to its own divine teleology. The laws of nature thus have a relationship to the divine law.

This is quite a different notion from teleological views which suggest that human behaviour is teleological, having happiness as its goal with this being gained through achieving pleasure or

---

[143] 'Teleological Notions in Biology', *The Stanford Encyclopaedia of Philosophy*, 2003, http://plato.stanford.edu/entries/teleology-biology/#ment (accessed 27 July 2011).

avoiding pain, or by achieving preference satisfaction. That kind of teleology is the basis for utilitarianism and some other forms of consequentialism which have the human being as their centre. In other words, they are anthropocentric and the environment is valued only insofar as protecting it is instrumentally necessary to achieve happiness. Against the charge of anthropocentrism some may argue, as Peter Singer has done, that happiness or preference satisfaction is not restricted to humans nor necessary for humans, but includes all those beings who can experience pleasure, pain or preference satisfaction; this includes some animals and excludes some humans.

This distinction in the understanding of teleology makes a significant difference. In respecting God's design, all creatures have a place, a purpose and a meaning for their existence and hence an intrinsic value. In the consequentialist approach they have only instrumental value, valued not in themselves but for their contribution to maximizing whatever it is – happiness, pleasure or satisfaction – that is achieved by their existence. In the consequentialist approach it is the states of affairs in the world that are the goal of morality. For a Christian who believes in creation, everything, including ourselves, has a divine purpose and meaning and we seek to act according to that divine purpose.

5.7 The Teleology of the Created Order

That we are created is of central importance to us and to our valuing each part of that creation according to its divine purpose. This has particular meaning in relation to ourselves because we understand that our capacities reflect the divine capacities of being the kind of being who can reason, doubt, question, affirm and love. In being able to love we are made in the divine image. Sin has a particular meaning for us because it is a rejection of the divine plan and thus involves us in turning away from the Creator. In sin we reject the very core of our being, the *imago Dei*, by turning away from who we are and why we exist; by turning away from loving God.

For each element of creation, intrinsic goodness has a particular meaning in relation to the divine plan. Its goodness is in its divine purpose and sin is the rejection of that essential goodness and purpose and hence a rejection of God. Morality for us, as believers in the Creator, is about accepting that divine purpose; thus it is not about states of affairs. The sin of Adam and Eve appears to be an offence involving the tree of knowledge; rather than accepting God's purposes for all of creation, they thought that they could determine good and evil for themselves.

Sin not only affected us; it affected all creation because it was a turning away from the meaning of all creation. It makes sense that this would generate confusion because humanity would no longer understand the meaning and purpose of each element of creation. Augustine explained the Fall in this way: thorns existed before the Fall. At the Fall man simply lost understanding of how to live and work around them. In sin we forget who we are; created beings who are utterly dependent on the Creator, not only for our moment by moment existence but also for the purpose and meaning of every aspect of the created order and the laws of nature that govern it. In losing that meaning, through the effects of sin, we surrender ourselves to the vicissitudes of meaninglessness and to the lack of purpose and order.

It is for this reason that Pope John Paul II referred to the fact that Christ came not only to redeem us, the sinners, but to redeem all of creation from the effects of our sin. In his 1991 Peace Day Message he wrote:

> At the conclusion of this Message, I should like to address directly my brothers and sisters in the Catholic Church, in order to remind them of their serious obligation to care

for all creation. The commitment of believers to a healthy environment for everyone stems directly from their belief in God the Creator, from their recognition of the effects of original and personal sin, and from the certainty of having been redeemed by Christ. Respect for life and for the dignity of the human person extends also to the rest of creation, which is called to join man in praising God (cf. Ps 148:96).

In *Veritatis Splendor,* Pope John Paul II writes:

> For mortal sin exists also when a person knowingly and willingly, for whatever reason, chooses something gravely disordered. In fact, such a choice already includes contempt for the divine law, a rejection of God's love for humanity and the whole of creation: the person turns away from God and loses charity. (n. 70)

At n. 73, he writes:

> ... the moral life has an essential *"teleological" character,* since it consists in the deliberate ordering of human acts to God, the supreme good and ultimate end *(telos)* of man. This is attested to once more by the question posed by the young man to Jesus: "What good must I do to have eternal life?". But this ordering to one's ultimate end is not something subjective, dependent solely upon one's intention. It presupposes that such acts are in themselves capable of being ordered to this end, insofar as they are in conformity with the authentic moral good of man, safeguarded by the commandments. This is what Jesus himself points out in his reply to the young man: "If you wish to enter into life, keep the commandments" (*Mt* 19:17).

The Second Vatican Council in *Gaudium et Spes,* gives a number of examples of intrinsically evil acts:

> Whatever is hostile to life itself, such as any kind of homicide, genocide, abortion, euthanasia and voluntary suicide; whatever violates the integrity of the human person, such as mutilation, physical and mental torture and attempts to coerce the spirit; whatever is offensive to human dignity, such as subhuman living conditions, arbitrary imprisonment, deportation, slavery, prostitution and trafficking in women and children; degrading conditions of work which treat labourers as mere instruments of profit, and not as free responsible persons: all these and the like are a disgrace, and so long as they infect human civilization they contaminate those who inflict them more than those who suffer injustice, and they are a negation of the honour due to the Creator.[144]

It could be said that this list contains offences against humanity but contains no list of offences against the rest of creation. However the document does say that such offences against humanity are a negation of the honour due to the Creator. Similarly, the Decalogue lists no offences against the rest of creation, just those against God and humanity.

An issue for a Christian environmental ethic is to find a place for defining a relationship between sin and the acts that cause disorder in the environment whereby the purposes for which each element of the created order exists have not been respected. As we have discussed, evolution provides us with an understanding of ecological balance and the natural purposes of each element. Turning away from God is what defines intrinsic evil. Destruction of the natural order acts against the divine purposes for each element of creation and thus constitutes a turning away from the Creator.

If, as discussed, we understand the Fall as loss of understanding

---

144 Second Vatican Council, *Gaudium et Spes*, op. cit., n. 27.

of creation and of the divine purposes intended for it then this readily explains for us the connection between sin and natural disorder and, hence, natural evils. What happens to us is a result of our loss of understanding, through sin, of how we might live harmoniously with our environment.

The intrinsic goodness of creation is that it reflects the purpose and design of the Creator; we sin when we choose to ignore His purposes and fail in our obligations to provide stewardship.

To the extent that Christianity focussed on offences against humanity and ignored offences against the rest of creation, our anthropocentrism was a failure to respect our relationship to God as Creator of all creation. That we are the pinnacle of creation gives us a special place which makes wilful destruction of human life a direct turning from God, but that does not mean the scope of our sinfulness is thereby exhausted. That God's goodness is reflected, also, in all creation requires us to seek to understand the rest of creation and to respect the purpose and design within it.

Alternatively, if we focus on the environment, and not the place of humanity within it, we can see human beings as a dreadful virus or a cancer on the universe, a spreading, migrating force for destruction and disorder.

An idea of the intrinsic goodness of all God's creation will seek harmony between human beings and the rest of creation, valuing the balance that exists within the created order and being able to be understood by humankind so that we can live with that harmony. We bring to it our own creativity, seeking to enhance this garden in which we have been placed but still respecting its natural beauty, balance and form. How we relate to one another and how we relate to the environment are linked in our appreciation of the natural created order and the evidence it provides of God's goodness that sustains us in being.

Pope Benedict XVI writes:

> The book of nature is one and indivisible: it takes in not only the environment but also life, sexuality, marriage, the family, social relations: in a word, integral human development. Our duties towards the environment are linked to our duties towards the human person, considered in himself and in relation to others. It would be wrong to uphold one set of duties while trampling on the other. Herein lies a grave contradiction in our mentality and practice today: one which demeans the person, disrupts the environment and damages society.[145]

---

145 Pope Benedict XVI, *Caritas in Veritate*, op. cit., n. 51.

6

THE GOODNESS OF ALL CREATION

6.1 The Environment and God's Love

Consider the following two basic moral questions: (1) What kinds of thing are intrinsically valuable, good or bad? (2) What makes an action right or wrong? Which prompts the question: Is there a link between them?

In our analysis of respect for human life we often read Christian thinkers who refer to the intrinsic worth or the inestimable worth of human life as the reason why killing a human being is wrong. Others will argue for the right to life on the basis that life is the most important of human rights because all other rights depend on us having life. The latter argument is based on claiming the instrumental rather than the intrinsic worth of a human life.

In the environment debate we face the issue of whether the rest of creation is valuable only because it is useful to human beings or whether it is intrinsically valuable. If a habitat, including all the creatures within it, was destroyed would that be a loss if it was in a wilderness which no human being visited and for which no-one had a use? Did God create the environment simply for human beings or did he create it for its own value? Is the universe important to God and not just as a temporary habitat for human beings?

Secondary to these questions is to ask whether the attribution of value to the environment means that the environment has rights, in the sense that damaging part of the environment would be wrong in itself and not just wrong because someone would lose the use, or other advantages, of it. Obviously we do not think so because we slaughter animals for food and cut down forests to build our homes. The argument tends to be about sustainability and whether the resources that we use are renewable, not about the intrinsic value of non human entities.

As Christians, the stepping off point, so to speak, on environmental issues is the notion that the environment is created by God and anything created by God is necessarily good.

From the Genesis 1 story there is a difference expressed between the elements of creation which are pronounced "good" and the creation of mankind which is pronounced "very good"; and that God has made us in His image and likeness. Immediately the question arises about the different status of humanity compared to the rest of creation.

In his Peace Day Message in 1991, Pope John Paul II explained that Adam and Eve were to have exercised their dominion over the earth (Gen 1:28) with wisdom and love. Instead, they destroyed the existing harmony by deliberately going against the Creator's plan, that is, by choosing to sin. He teaches that Jesus redeemed not just us but all Creation:

> Christians believe that the Death and Resurrection of Christ accomplished the work of reconciling humanity to the Father, who "was pleased ... through (Christ) to reconcile to himself ALL THINGS, whether on earth or in heaven, making peace by the blood of his cross" (Col. 1:19-20). Creation was thus made new (cf. Rev. 21:5). Once subjected to the bondage of sin and decay (cf. Rom. 8:21), it has now received new life while "we wait for new heavens and a new earth in which righteousness dwells" (2 Pt 3:13). Thus, the Father "has made known to us in all wisdom and insight the mystery ... which he set forth

in Christ as a plan for the fullness of time, to unite ALL THINGS in him, all things in heaven and things on earth" (Eph. 1:9-10).[146]

The Pope spoke of the lack of respect for life as underlying the ecological problem; in this regard he argued for respect for the ecology because ecological balance is needed to preserve human life. Economic interests should not take priority over the good of individuals. Pollution or environmental destruction is the result of an unnatural and reductionist vision which at times leads to contempt for man. He also spoke of the disturbance of ecological balances by the uncontrolled destruction of animal and plant life or by a reckless exploitation of natural resources to mankind's disadvantage. Finally, he referred to the biological disturbance that could result from indiscriminate genetic manipulation and from the unscrupulous development of new forms of plant and animal life, to say nothing of unacceptable experimentation regarding the origins of human life itself, all of which would lead mankind to the very threshold of self-destruction.[147]

In other words, Pope John Paul II addressed the environmental issues in terms of the effect of damage to the environment on human beings, implying that the value of the environment is instrumental rather than intrinsic. It is only mankind that has intrinsic value, inherent dignity and, hence, equal and inalienable rights.

St Thomas Aquinas also held that all creation is good because it is made by God and therefore must be good. However he does not conclude therefore that damaging or destroying animals, plants, mountains, forests or oceans would be necessarily a bad thing to do. He takes the view that only human beings have that status and that other forms of nature only need to be protected insofar as they serve human interests. For Thomas, cruelty to animals is

---

146 Pope John Paul II, *Peace with God the Creator, Peace with All Creation*, op. cit., n. 4.
147 Ibid.

only wrong because it may predispose a human being to be cruel to human beings. Forests exist for the benefit of human beings; for wood, for building, for fuel and for the pleasure their beauty gives us. Thus for St Thomas it is only human beings who are intrinsically good. The rest of creation is good but only instrumentally in order to serve the needs and desires of humanity.

In the Old Testament the Jews were forbidden to muzzle the ox that treads out the corn (Deuteronomy 25:4) or to yoke together an ox and an ass (Deuteronomy 22:10). In Proverbs it is written, "The just regardeth the lives of his beasts: but the bowels of the wicked are cruel" (Proverbs 12:10).

Interpreting these passages, St Thomas defends taking the life of an animal but prohibits cruelty towards brutes because this may lead to cruelty towards men: acknowledging only that "because an injury to brutes may result in loss to the owner, or on account of some symbolic signification".[148] In other words, he does not condemn cruelty to animals in itself, but only because of its effect on the perpetrator and the likelihood that cruelty or, alternatively, pity for animals would extend to other human beings. In the *Summa Theologica* he writes:

> But if man's affection be one of passion, then it is moved also in regard to other animals: for since the passion of pity is caused by the afflictions of others; and since it happens that even irrational animals are sensible to pain, it is possible for the affection of pity to arise in a man with regard to the sufferings of animals. Now it is evident that if a man practice a pitiful affection for animals, he is all the more disposed to take pity on his fellow-men: wherefore it is written (Proverbs 11:10): "The just regardeth the lives of his beasts: but the bowels of the wicked are cruel." Consequently the Lord, in order to inculcate pity to the

---

148 Aquinas, *Summa Contra Gentiles*, Bk. 2, Chapter 112.

Jewish people, who were prone to cruelty, wished them to practice pity even with regard to dumb animals, and forbade them to do certain things savoring of cruelty to animals.[149]

Thomas argues that human beings have moral worth because we have an immortal soul and thus a teleology to be with God in eternity. For Thomas, God is in no way dependent upon us. He loves us with a love that is agapeic. It is disinterested love unaffected by what we might do or think. He loves us for our own sake because we are made in His image and likeness and He wants us to flourish according to the rational nature that He created for us. For St Thomas, no other species has an immortal rational soul and so no other species has a teleology with God in eternity. On Aquinas's account the rest of the material universe exists only for a time and has no purpose beyond that time. This view thus places humanity in a completely different category, one of being loved by God for all eternity.

One of the puzzles for us is the claim that Pope Benedict makes in *Deus Caritas Est* that God not only loves us, He also wants to be loved by us. The Pope refers to this as *Eros*. This is something of a challenge for St Thomas. Of God's love, St Thomas writes that God's love is not passionate,[150] that God loves all things equally and that his love is different from our love because God's will is the cause of Goodness. Goodness in things and in persons calls forth our will and when we love something we will goodness to it: whereas the love of God infuses and creates goodness. St Thomas argues that God's love is not passionate because passion is something that belongs to being embodied:

> The cognitive faculty does not move except through the medium of the appetitive: and just as in ourselves

---
149 Aquinas, *Summa Theologica II:I*, Q. 102.
150 Aquinas, *Summa Theologica I*, Q. 20.

the universal reason moves through the medium of the particular reason, as stated in De Anima iii, 58,75, so in ourselves the intellectual appetite, or the will as it is called, moves through the medium of the sensitive appetite. Hence, in us the sensitive appetite is the proximate motive-force of our bodies. Some bodily change therefore always accompanies an act of the sensitive appetite, and this change affects especially the heart, which, as the Philosopher says (De part. animal. iii, 4), is the first principle of movement in animals. Therefore acts of the sensitive appetite, inasmuch as they have annexed to them some bodily change, are called passions; whereas acts of the will are not so called. Love, therefore, and joy and delight are passions; in so far as they denote acts of the intellective appetite, they are not passions. It is in this latter sense that they are in God. Hence the Philosopher says (Ethic. vii): "God rejoices by an operation that is one and simple," and for the same reason He loves without passion.[151]

On the matter of God's love for creation and His love for human beings, St Thomas writes:

Friendship cannot exist except towards rational creatures, who are capable of returning love, and communicating one with another in the various works of life, and who may fare well or ill, according to the changes of fortune and happiness; even as to them is benevolence properly speaking exercised. But irrational creatures cannot attain to loving God, nor to any share in the intellectual and beatific life that He lives. Strictly speaking, therefore, God does not love irrational creatures with the love of friendship; but as it were with the love of desire, in so far as He orders them to rational creatures, and even to

---

151 Ibid.

Himself. Yet this is not because He stands in need of them; but only on account of His goodness, and of the services they render to us. For we can desire a thing for others as well as for ourselves.[152]

On the other hand St Thomas writes of the angels as having self love. He writes: "Angels like men by nature strive for their own good and their own perfection, and this means loving themselves."[153]

Heather Erb argues that St Thomas' notion of divine love is impersonal and therefore unmeritorious.[154] She argues otherwise, that God's love includes a desire for friendship with us. It is a relationship in which our love for God plays a part. It is therefore inclusive of *eros* in the way in which Pope Benedict has defined the latter. Love of friendship is part of the desire for the universal good, God Himself.

Thus there would seem to be a tension between St Thomas' view of God's love for us, which is dispassionate and disinterested, and Pope Benedict's view that *eros* is also part of Divine love. That is to say that God wants to be loved by us and that the love that Jesus expressed desired friendship. At Gethsemane he wanted the apostles to be with him. He cried when he heard that Lazarus had died. In the parables of the prodigal son and of the shepherd, which we understand were meant to display the love of the Father, love for the lost one is passionate and desirous of their return.

The notion that God does not need us leads St Thomas to recognize only agapeic love in God and not eros. This is in clear contrast to what Pope Benedict writes:

---

152 Ibid.
153 Ibid, Q. 60, Art. 3.
154 Heather Erb, 'From Rivulets to the Fountain's Source: Image and Love in Aquinas' Christian Anthropology', in P.A. Pagan Aguiar and T. Auer (eds.), *The Human Person and a Culture of Freedom*, Washington, Catholic University Press, 2009, p. 87.

> The one God in whom Israel believes, on the other hand, loves with a personal love. His love, moreover, is an elective love: among all the nations he chooses Israel and loves her – but he does so precisely with a view to healing the whole human race. God loves, and his love may certainly be called *eros*, yet it is also totally *agape*.[155]

The Pope continues this theme in the next section saying:

> The philosophical dimension to be noted in this biblical vision, and its importance from the standpoint of the history of religions, lies in the fact that on the one hand we find ourselves before a strictly metaphysical image of God: God is the absolute and ultimate source of all being; but this universal principle of creation – the *Logos*, primordial reason – is at the same time a lover with all the passion of a true love. *Eros* is thus supremely ennobled, yet at the same time it is so purified as to become one with *agape*.[156]

In his analysis of the New Testament he pursues this notion that God's love is both giving of Himself and wanting to be loved by us:

> This divine activity now takes on dramatic form when, in Jesus Christ, it is God himself who goes in search of the "stray sheep", a suffering and lost humanity. When Jesus speaks in his parables of the shepherd who goes after the lost sheep, of the woman who looks for the lost coin, of the father who goes to meet and embrace his prodigal son, these are no mere words: they constitute an explanation of his very being and activity. His death on the Cross is the culmination of that turning of God against himself in which he gives himself in order to raise man up and save

---

[155] Pope Benedict XVI, *Deus Caritas Est*, 25 December 2005, n. 9, http://w2.vatican.va/content/benedict-xvi/en/encyclicals/documents/hf_ben-xvi_enc_20051225_deus-caritas-est.html (accessed 2010-2014).
[156] Ibid., n. 10.

him. This is love in its most radical form. By contemplating the pierced side of Christ (cf. 19:37), we can understand the starting-point of this Encyclical Letter: "God is love" (*1 Jn* 4:8). It is there that this truth can be contemplated. It is from there that our definition of love must begin. In this contemplation the Christian discovers the path along which his life and love must move.[157]

He makes the same point in relation to marriage:

> First, *eros* is somehow rooted in man's very nature; Adam is a seeker, who "abandons his mother and father" in order to find woman; only together do the two represent complete humanity and become "one flesh". The second aspect is equally important. From the standpoint of creation, *eros* directs man towards marriage, to a bond which is unique and definitive; thus, and only thus, does it fulfil its deepest purpose. Corresponding to the image of a monotheistic God is monogamous marriage. Marriage based on exclusive and definitive love becomes the icon of the relationship between God and his people and vice versa. God's way of loving becomes the measure of human love. This close connection between *eros* and marriage in the Bible has practically no equivalent in extra-biblical literature.[158]

St Augustine writes of the nature of God's love for us as emotional love:

> Wherefore even the Lord Himself, when He condescended to lead a human life in the form of a slave, had no sin whatever, and yet exercised these emotions where He judged they should be exercised. For as there was in Him a true human body and a true human soul, so was there

---

157 Ibid., n. 11.
158 Ibid., n. 10.

also a true human emotion. When, therefore, we read in the Gospel that the hard-heartedness of the Jews moved Him to sorrowful indignation, Mark 3:5 that He said, I am glad for your sakes, to the intent ye may believe, John 11:15 that when about to raise Lazarus He even shed tears, John 11:35 that He earnestly desired to eat the passover with His disciples, Luke 22:15 that as His passion drew near His soul was sorrowful, Matthew 26:38 these emotions are certainly not falsely ascribed to Him. But as He became man when it pleased Him, so, in the grace of His definite purpose, when it pleased Him He experienced those emotions in His human soul.[159]

The significance for all creation, of us being both *agape* and *eros*, is that our relationship to God is different from His relationship to animals precisely because we are able to love Him, able to form a friendship with Him. Our existence has an enduring purpose in the Creator's design, to love Him and be loved by Him.

One way of seeing God's relationship to all creation is to see His love for humankind, the pinnacle of all creation. The notion that we have evolved from animals increases that sense of our connectedness to the rest of creation. God's love for all creation is for the creation that has yielded humanity in His image and likeness. His friendship with humanity is thus a friendship with all creation. We come to the Father through Christ and all creation comes to Christ through humanity. We are, in that sense, the mediators of God's love to all creation through our capacity to love. In that capacity is our lovableness to God, and therefore, since we are part of it, the lovableness of all creation that resulted in humanity.

The attribution of the word *eros* to God by Pope Benedict is challenging. The Greek word *eros* is ambiguous. In the Platonic

---

[159] St Augustine, *City of God*, bk. 14, chapter 9.

dialogues, it encompasses affection enkindled by physical beauty, passionate joy, intoxicated god-sent madness, the impulse to philosophical contemplation of the world and existence and the exaltation that went with the contemplation of divine beauty. The link between love and joy seems to be particularly strong in Plato's understanding of *eros*.[160] In attributing *eros* to God, Pope Benedict attributes passion:

> Hosea above all shows us that this *agape* dimension of God's love for man goes far beyond the aspect of gratuity. Israel has committed "adultery" and has broken the covenant; God should judge and repudiate her. It is precisely at this point that God is revealed to be God and not man: "How can I give you up, O Ephraim! How can I hand you over, O Israel! ... My heart recoils within me, my compassion grows warm and tender. I will not execute my fierce anger, I will not again destroy Ephraim; for I am God and not man, the Holy One in your midst" (*Hos* 11:8-9). God's passionate love for his people – for humanity – is at the same time a forgiving love.[161]

By His love God wills us to be for our own sakes. He also wishes the rest of creation to be, or else it would not be. But our tradition has it that He only wishes it to be for the uses that it has for us and, therefore, he gives us dominion over it (Genesis 1:28).

The goodness of creation is thus essentially instrumental but our dominion is a stewardship not an ownership. Our environment is governed by the laws of nature and it ill-behoves us to not understand what those laws are. We need to understand them so that we can live in ecological balance with our environment.

In 1991, Pope John Paul II wrote:

> The gradual depletion of the ozone layer and the related

---

160 Josef Pieper, *Faith, Hope, Love*, Chicago, Ignatius Press, 1992, pp. 155-156.
161 Pope Benedict XVI, *Deus Caritas Est*, op. cit., n. 10.

"greenhouse effect" has now reached crisis proportions as a consequence of industrial growth, massive urban concentrations and vastly increased energy needs. Industrial waste, the burning of fossil fuels, unrestricted deforestation, the use of certain types of herbicides, coolants and propellants: all of these are known to harm the atmosphere and environment. The resulting meteorological and atmospheric changes range from damage to health to the possible future submersion of low-lying lands.

While in some cases the damage already done may well be irreversible, in many other cases it can still be halted. It is necessary, however, that the entire human community – individuals, States and international bodies – take seriously the responsibility that is theirs.[162]

6.2 Christianity and Anthropocentrism

Despite the recent efforts by Pope Paul VI, Pope John Paul II and Pope Benedict XVI to insist upon our obligations to the environment, Christianity is often held, by environmentalists, to be accountable for an anthropocentric and hence exploitative attitude to the environment:

> Especially in its Western form, Christianity is the most anthropocentric religion the world has seen. As early as the second century both Tertullian and Saint Irenaeus of Lyons were insisting that when God shaped Adam he was foreshadowing the image of the incarnate Christ, the Second Adam. Man shares, in great measure, God's transcendence of nature. Christianity, in absolute contrast to ancient paganism and Asia's religions (except, perhaps, Zorastrianism), not only established a dualism of man

---

[162] Pope John Paul II, *Peace with God the Creator, Peace with All Creation*, op. cit., n. 4.

and nature but also insisted that it is God's will that man exploit nature for his proper ends.[163]

Concern for the environment was expressed very briefly by Pope Paul VI when he wrote in the Apostolic Letter *Octogesima Adveniens*:

> While the horizon of man is thus being modified according to the images that are chosen for him, another transformation is making itself felt, one which is the dramatic and unexpected consequence of human activity. Man is suddenly becoming aware that by an ill-considered exploitation of nature he risks destroying it and becoming in his turn the victim of this degradation. Not only is the material environment becoming a permanent menace – pollution and refuse, new illness and absolute destructive capacity – but the human framework is no longer under man's control, thus creating an environment for tomorrow which may well be intolerable. This is a wide-ranging social problem which concerns the entire human family.
>
> The Christian must turn to these new perceptions in order to take on responsibility, together with the rest of men, for a destiny which from now on is shared by all.[164]

In *Centesimus Annus*, Pope John Paul II wrote:

> Equally worrying is *the ecological question* which accompanies the problem of consumerism and which is closely connected to it. In his desire to have and to enjoy rather than to be and to grow, man consumes the resources of the earth and his own life in an excessive and disordered way. At the root of the senseless destruction

---

163 Lynn White Jr., *The Historical Roots of Our Ecological Crisis*, http://www.zbi.ee/~kalevi/lwhite.htm (accessed 2010-2014).
164 Pope Paul VI, *Octogesima Adveniens*, 14 May 1971, n. 21, http://www.vatican.va/holy_father/paul_vi/apost_letters/documents/hf_p-vi_apl_19710514_octogesima-adveniens_en.html (accessed 2010-2014).

of the natural environment lies an anthropological error, which unfortunately is widespread in our day. Man, who discovers his capacity to transform and in a certain sense create the world through his own work, forgets that this is always based on God's prior and original gift of the things that are. Man thinks that he can make arbitrary use of the earth, subjecting it without restraint to his will, as though it did not have its own requisites and a prior God-given purpose, which man can indeed develop but must not betray. Instead of carrying out his role as a co-operator with God in the work of creation, man sets himself up in place of God and thus ends up provoking a rebellion on the part of nature, which is more tyrannized than governed by him.

In all this, one notes first the poverty or narrowness of man's outlook, motivated as he is by a desire to possess things rather than to relate them to the truth, and lacking that disinterested, unselfish and aesthetic attitude that is born of wonder in the presence of being and of the beauty which enables one to see in visible things the message of the invisible God who created them. In this regard, humanity today must be conscious of its duties and obligations towards future generations.[165]

Benedict XVI, in his 2010 Peace Day message, *If You Want to Cultivate Peace, Protect Creation*, wrote:

Can we remain indifferent before the problems associated with such realities as climate change, desertification, the deterioration and loss of productivity in vast agricultural areas, the pollution of rivers and aquifers, the loss of biodiversity, the increase of natural catastrophes and the deforestation of equatorial and tropical regions? Can we disregard the growing phenomenon of 'environmental refugees', people who are forced by the degradation

---

165 Pope John Paul II, *Centesimus Annus*, 1 May 1991.

of their natural habitat to forsake it – and often their possessions as well – in order to face the dangers and uncertainties of forced displacement?

Highlighting that these environmental problems are intricately linked to the world's current economic model, the Pope called for a "a profound, long-term review of our model of development, one which would take into consideration the meaning of the economy and its goals with an eye to correcting its malfunctions and misapplications."[166]

However despite these present day messages, Christianity has been accused of applying the Genesis 1:28 passage, "And God blessed them. And God said to them, "Be fruitful and multiply and fill the earth and subdue it and have dominion over the fish of the sea and over the birds of the heavens and over every living thing that moves on the earth,"" in such a way as to regard the environment as open to exploitation.

Environmental philosopher Paul W. Taylor[167] argues against anthropocentrism. He argues instead for a biocentric view of environmental ethics in which we should respect every living organism. He contrasts this with views, such as those of Peter Singer,[168] that argue for protecting those who have sentience, and with Christianity which considers humanity alone to be intrinsically valuable.

Some environmentalists place their emphasis on the worth of ecosystems and species within them. This was argued as early

---

166 Pope Benedict XVI, *If You Want to Cultivate Peace, Protect Creation*, 1 January 2010, http://www.vatican.va/holy_father/benedict_xvi/messages/peace/documents/hf_ben-xvi_mes_20091208_xliii-world-day-peace_en.html (accessed 2010-2014).
167 P. W. Taylor, *Respect for Nature: A Theory of Environmental Ethics*, Princeton University Press, 1986.
168 Peter Singer (ed.), *In Defense of Animals: The Second Wave*, Oxford, Blackwell, 2005.

as 1948 by Aldo Leopold.[169] There are also those who argue for biodiversity as an intrinsic good.[170] Thus any loss of a species would be a great evil.

Taylor, on the other hand, argues for the value of each individual life. Taylor thinks individualism follows from biocentrism, as only individuals are alive and all living organisms, including humans, have equal inherent worth.

According to Taylor, human beings enjoy no specially privileged place within the earth's community of life. He argues that humans are contingent, biological beings and share with other organisms the biological requirements for life that are not completely under our control. We are equally vulnerable. We share with them an inability to guarantee the fundamental conditions of our existence. In many respects, and importantly, humans are creatures of forces we do not control.

He argues that we have the same status as other life forms because we share the same origin as other creatures and so have ties of kinship with them. The earth's life processes (evolution) brought all of us into existence; knowing how they came to be is knowing how we came to exist as well. Further we are recent arrivals: the earth was "teeming with life" long before we arrived and when we did, we entered a place in which others had resided for hundreds of millions of years. Finally we are not the ultimate purpose of natural processes. He argues that the idea that humans are the final goal of the evolutionary process is absurd; it's as if the rest of nature was waiting on our arrival and applauded when we finally appeared. Importantly, we depend on other species: humans

---

169 Aldo Leopold, *A Sand County Almanac*, New York, Oxford University Press, 1949.
170 Anup Shah, 'Why Is Biodiversity Important? Who Cares?', *Global Issues*, 2009, http://www.globalissues.org/article/170/why-is-biodiversity-important-who-cares (accessed 2 Dec 2010).

are absolutely dependent on other forms of life; without them we would cease to exist. We are needy dependents on the fabric of life around us. Other species don't depend on us: life on this planet is not dependent on us; in fact, often it would do much better without us.

Taylor also argues that the natural world is an interdependent system, the basic insight of the science of ecology. He recognises a teleology in all life forms: all organisms and only organisms are goal-directed centres of life that have goods of their own and hence welfare interests that we can morally consider for their own sake. Organisms have a (non-subjective) "point of view" that we can adopt by judging events as good or bad depending on whether the organisms are benefitted or harmed.

Against Peter Singer, he argues that having preference interests, conscious desires or wants is not necessary for being morally considerable. Thus insentient organisms including plants, fungi, microbes, and many invertebrate animals should be included. Having welfare interests is thus a necessary condition for being morally considerable. If a being doesn't have a good of its own, then there is nothing to morally consider; no "point of view" to adopt. It can't be benefited or harmed; it has no welfare we could protect. Thus stones or piles of sand have no moral value of their own. They are only instrumentally valuable. Nonliving natural entities including species, ecosystems, and biological/geological entities and processes are thus also not morally considerable, since they too have no good of their own.

On those grounds Taylor argues that anthropocentrism is an unjustified bias: we should be a species that is impartial and egalitarian because to argue that humans are superior, because we have capacities non-humans lack such as moral agency, ignores the fact that other species have capacities that we lack such as the ability to photosynthesize, to live 10,000 years, to produce

20 million offspring or to regenerate oneself after being put in a blender. To argue that humans are superior because our capacities are more valuable, such as the ability to do mathematics compared to a monkey's ability to climb a tree, is to judge illegitimately the value of capacities from the perspective of what is good for human life. From the perspective of what is good in a monkey's life, tree climbing ability is of greater value. He draws a parallel between the views of the nobility in the Middle Ages who believed that they were superior to peasants and the Christian view that human beings are superior.

The Taylor analysis is excessive in its disregard of the significance of intelligence and the human capacities to doubt, wonder, affirm and above all love. However there are some elements of it that are challenging. If we accept that human beings have evolved then it is true that we are in kinship with the rest of creation. Even abiding by the literal story of Genesis we are still made by the same Creator and the rest of creation, like us, reflects its Divine Designer.

6.3 The Goodness of Creation

Without going as far as Paul Taylor, Peter Singer, Aldo Leopold or Anup Shah in their views about the importance of other life forms or ecologies, we can see, from the perspective of the potential harm to us and to future generations, the importance of the environment and the need for us to take good care of it. From a Christian anthropocentric perspective, we can see that not taking care of the environment and not respecting the laws of nature, which determine the survival of our environment, are harmful to us.

However, there is a further question to be asked concerning the moral status of the environment and the sub-human creatures within it. Clearly, human beings with our capacity to form a friendship with God occupy a different place in God's love from the rest of creation. Nevertheless, the Genesis story declares each element of our environment to be *good* and St Thomas declares that all creation is good, being made by God. In many ways, St Augustine could be considered the patron saint of the environment because he saw it not just as useful but as expressive of the Creator:

> Behold, the heaven and earth are; they proclaim that they were made, for they are changed and varied. Whereas whatsoever hath not been made, and yet hath being, hath nothing in it which there was not before; this is what it is to be changed and varied. They also proclaim that they made not themselves; "therefore we are, because we have been made; we were not therefore before we were, so that we could have made ourselves." And the voice of those that speak is in itself an evidence. Thou, therefore, Lord, didst make these things; Thou who art beautiful, for they are beautiful; Thou who art good, for they are good; Thou who art, for they are. Nor even so are they beautiful, nor good, nor are they, as Thou their Creator art; compared with whom they are neither beautiful, nor good, nor are at all. These things we know, thanks be to Thee. And our knowledge, compared with Thy knowledge, is ignorance.[171]

This does raise a question about whether, from a Christian perspective, more should be said about the environment other than that that it is instrumentally valuable and essential for our own survival.

Rev. Dr. George Cairns of the Iona Community in Scotland thinks that modern Christianity has lost meaning. He writes:

> What we have lost is participative consciousness, which understands that our lives are profoundly related to the

---

[171] St Augustine, *Confessions*, bk. 11, chapter 4, retrieved from http://www.leaderu.com/cyber/books/augconfessions/bk11.html#BOOKXICHAPI (accessed 2010-2014).

physical, mental and spiritual aspects of all of creation. Another way of putting this is that we are completely relational beings. Reconnection with all of creation as sacred and responsive and alive is our great task in the early 21st century.[172]

There is a parallel here with the concept that Pope John Paul II used in *Veritatis Splendor* referring to "participated theonomy". He rejected saying that "obedience to God as a heteronomy, in which human beings are subject to the will of something all-powerful, absolute, extraneous to man and intolerant of his freedom". "Such a heteronomy would be nothing but a form of alienation, contrary to divine wisdom and to the dignity of the human person."[173] A heteronomy of that kind is often described as fundamentalist. However the pope also rejected an autonomy by which we create our own morality as that "would be in contradiction to the Revelation of the Covenant and of the redemptive Incarnation."[174]

He went on to say:

> Others speak, and rightly so, of *theonomy,* or *participated theonomy,* since man's free obedience to God's law effectively implies that human reason and human will participate in God's wisdom and providence. By forbidding man to "eat of the tree of the knowledge of good and evil", God makes it clear that man does not originally possess such "knowledge" as something properly his own, but only participates in it by the light of natural reason and of Divine Revelation, which manifest to him the requirements and the promptings of eternal wisdom.

---

172 G. Cairns, 'Celtic Christianity Homily: The Goodness of Creation', delivered at the Union Community Church in Valparaiso, Indiana, 3 May 2009, http://wn.com/celtic_christianity_homily_the_goodness_of_creation_by_rev_dr_george_cairns (accessed 2010-2014).
173 Pope John Paul II, *Veritatis Splendor*, n. 36.
174 Ibid.

> Law must therefore be considered an expression of divine wisdom: by submitting to the law, freedom submits to the truth of creation. Consequently one must acknowledge in the freedom of the human person the image and the nearness of God, who is present in all (cf. *Eph* 4:6). But one must likewise acknowledge the majesty of the God of the universe and revere the holiness of the law of God, who is infinitely transcendent: *Deus semper maior*.[175]

Our obedience to the Divine Law involves a law which is inclusive of us, with which we are involved because we are made in the Creator's image and can choose to strive to be like Him. This is a central theme of the theology of the body, of what has become known as Trinitarian anthropology. In baptism we are called to be a witness to God's love, a God whose love is evident in the life, suffering and death of Christ, but also in all creation. Through our free obedience in loving God and loving His commandments we participate in the law not as the passive recipients of an arbitrary, alienated law imposed upon us, but a law that implies that human reason and human will participate in God's wisdom and providence as Pope John Paul expressed it. By being close to and loving all creation we love the Creator and through this we can develop in understanding of Him.

Pope Benedict writes in *Deus Caritas Est* about all creation being dear to God:

> ... There is only one God, the Creator of heaven and earth, who is thus the God of all. Two facts are significant about this statement: all other gods are not God, and the universe in which we live has its source in God and was created by him. Certainly, the notion of creation is found elsewhere, yet only here does it become absolutely clear that it is not one god among many, but the one true God

---

[175] Ibid.

himself who is the source of all that exists; the whole world comes into existence by the power of his creative Word. Consequently, his creation is dear to him, for it was willed by him and "made" by him.[176]

In his encyclical *Caritas in Veritate* he writes of the importance of respecting the environment as God's creation:

> When nature, including the human being, is viewed as the result of mere chance or evolutionary determinism, our sense of responsibility wanes. In nature, the believer recognizes the wonderful result of God's creative activity, which we may use responsibly to satisfy our legitimate needs, material or otherwise, while respecting the intrinsic balance of creation. If this vision is lost, we end up either considering nature an untouchable taboo or, on the contrary, abusing it. Neither attitude is consonant with the Christian vision of nature as the fruit of God's creation.
>
> *Nature expresses a design of love and truth.* It is prior to us, and it has been given to us by God as the setting for our life. Nature speaks to us of the Creator (cf. Rom 1:20) and his love for humanity. It is destined to be "recapitulated" in Christ at the end of time (cf. Eph 1:9-10; Col 1:19-20). Thus it too is a "vocation". Nature is at our disposal not as "a heap of scattered refuse", but as a gift of the Creator who has given it an inbuilt order, enabling man to draw from it the principles needed in order "to till it and keep it" (Gen 2:15).[177]

In his Peace Day Message in 2010 referred to previously, Pope Benedict quotes Psalm 8: "When I look at your heavens, the work of your hands, the moon and the stars which you have established; what is man that you are mindful of him, and the son of man that

---

176 Pope Benedict XVI, *Deus Caritas Est*, op. cit., n. 9.
177 Pope Benedict XVI, *Caritas in Veritate*, op. cit., n. 48.

you care for him?" (Ps 8:4-5). Then he refers to Dante's poem where he claims that contemplating the beauty of creation inspires us to recognize the love of the Creator, that Love which "moves the sun and the other stars".[178]

The Pope concludes his Message with the words:

> If you want to cultivate peace, protect creation. The quest for peace by people of good will surely would become easier if all acknowledge the indivisible relationship between God, human beings and the whole of creation. In the light of divine Revelation and in fidelity to the Church's Tradition, Christians have their own contribution to make. They contemplate the cosmos and its marvels in light of the creative work of the Father and the redemptive work of Christ, who by his death and resurrection has reconciled with God "all things, whether on earth or in heaven" (Col 1:20). Christ, crucified and risen, has bestowed his Spirit of holiness upon mankind, to guide the course of history in anticipation of that day when, with the glorious return of the Saviour, there will be "new heavens and a new earth" (2 Pet 3:13), in which justice and peace will dwell for ever. Protecting the natural environment in order to build a world of peace is thus a duty incumbent upon each and all. It is an urgent challenge, one to be faced with renewed and concerted commitment; it is also a providential opportunity to hand down to coming generations the prospect of a better future for all.

There is more to creation than just utility. In being the work of the Creator, like humankind our environment also displays the divine nature. In the great marvels and the complexity of nature we can see His wisdom and insight. As human beings we stand physically and spiritually in relationship with all creation because

---
178 Dante Alighieri, *The Divine Comedy*, Paradiso: Canto XXXIII, 145.

we come from the same source. When Christ came to redeem us from the effects of sin he came to redeem all creation. It is sin that dominates and exploits our environment. In Christ we have the opportunity to seek peace in communion with the Creator, peace with God, peace with all creation.[179]

---

[179] Pope John Paul II, *Peace with God the Creator, Peace with All Creation*, op. cit.

7

THE BEAUTY OF ALL CREATION

7.1 Introduction

In this chapter, the role of beauty or aesthetic appreciation within Christian philosophy and theology is considered as a way into the consideration of the importance, to us, of natural phenomena. We can think of the environment in terms of our physical dependence upon it, the human causes of environmental degradation and the danger to future generations because of pollution, climate change, rising seas, increased floods, droughts, fires and the loss of non-renewable resources. But in considering our relationship to God, there is much more to the environment than our physical dependence upon it.

All creation bears the imprint of the mind that created it. In the beauty of the world around us we can see evidence of the mind of God. We need no instruction to appreciate the beauty of a sunset or a rainbow, a forest or a mountainside, the breathtaking sights of a coral reef, or a condor in flight, a lion or an elephant in their natural habitat. An issue for philosophers and theologians, then, is how do we come to possess this knowledge of what is beautiful and what is this knowledge. For post-moderns there is no such knowledge. In their view when I say something is beautiful I am doing no more than expressing the feelings of pleasure and the approval that it invokes in me. However, idealists such as Plato and Kant saw appreciation of beauty as a kind of knowing. Hans Urs von Balthasar goes further and rejects the idea of transcendentals as a category of knowing that can be defined and separated from each other, seeing them instead as the properties or determinants of being that permeate all aspects of our being. Particularly interesting in this discussion are the relationships between goodness, truth and beauty. Can the beautiful be false or depraved? In the Christian tradition the response would be negative, precisely because the transcendentals are interrelated. By being aspects of the divine being they are interrelated.

In relation to appreciating our environment, the relationship of beauty to truth and goodness is an important issue. The postmodern view, that there is nothing objective in the appreciation of beauty, condemns us to an anthropocentric idea of natural beauty, simply that which gives us pleasure. Nothing is beautiful in itself.

The Early Fathers puzzled over the place of beauty in the scheme of things. Was Jesus handsome? Is it important that we think of him as so? What does it mean to say that he is beautiful? Is there a connection between goodness and beauty? Is the beauty of Jesus the beauty of His infinite goodness; and thus evident even in the beaten, bruised and tortured face that would have confronted Pilate and the crowds that cried out to have him executed?

7.2 Augustine, Idealism and the Transcendentals

The debates over aesthetic judgment and moral judgment are similar and to some extent connected. Like truth and goodness, beauty is considered by idealists to be one of the transcendentals. That is to say it is one of those things which lies beyond the limits of experience and has more to do with our being than to do with empirical knowledge. We make judgments which do not come from experience, but, nevertheless, are legitimately applied to the data or contents of knowledge furnished by experience.[180] This is

---

180 Immanuel Kant, *The Critique of Judgement, Part I: Critique of Aesthetic Judgement*, trans. J.C. Meredith, retrieved from http://ebooks.adelaide.edu.au/k/kant/immanuel/k16j/ (accessed 29 Dec 2010).

what is meant by *a priori* judgments. Theologically it is the idea that, in being made in God's image and likeness, we are given an innate knowledge of the transcendentals. Because we are made in the image and likeness of God we can appreciate beauty, just as we can appreciate truth and goodness. The transcendentals, in being beyond empirical knowledge, are to do with the nature of our being as the *imago Dei*.

Plato refers to this as *anamnesis*. Believing that knowledge of the transcendentals is already possessed by the student, he sees the role of a teacher, in that respect, being more like a midwife bringing to the consciousness of the student knowledge that the student already possesses. In his dialogue, called the *Meno*,[181] he has Socrates question a slave boy about geometry. The slave boy is led to produce the right answer by being questioned rather than being instructed. In the *Phaedo* he has Socrates say:

> For this is clear, that when we perceived something, either by the help of sight or hearing, or some other sense, there was no difficulty in receiving from this a conception of some other thing like or unlike which had been forgotten and which was associated with this; and therefore, as I was saying, one of two alternatives follows: either we had this knowledge at birth, and continued to know through life; or, after birth, those who are said to learn only remember, and learning is recollection only.[182]

For Plato, and for Immanuel Kant, knowledge of beauty is something that we possess innately, inherently. For Plato, beauty is determined according to an idea of beauty that we already possess and then apply to experience. This notion of pre-existent

---
[181] Plato, *Meno*, trans. B. Jowett, retrieved from http://www.fullbooks.com/Meno.html (accessed 2010-2014).
[182] Plato, *Phaedo*, trans. B. Jowett, retrieved from http://classics.mit.edu/Plato/phaedo.html (accessed 2010-2014).

ideas by which we understand the world is called Plato's Theory of Forms. The world around us contains structures or elements, like roundness or colour, that we already know as ideas which we then recognize. For Plato, beauty is one of those pre-existing ideas. However, for a Christian we understand that this knowledge, this way of perceiving comes from God and that beauty is related to truth and goodness and is part of our being.

Our particular interest in this subject is the connection between the transcendental of beauty as it applies to creation and the goodness of creation and, therefore, its intrinsic worth, and its vocational importance in our relationship to God. A sound environmental ethic will include an understanding of creation and therefore the beauty and intrinsic worth of all created things. I include Kant in this analysis because he has something philosophically interesting to say about beauty that challenges post-modernism and, like Augustine, Aquinas, Plato and Aristotle, explores it not as empirical knowledge but still as a kind of knowing. There is a difference between Plato, Augustine and Kant, who understand that the perception of beauty is a result of anamnesis, that is to say they hold that the capacity to perceive beauty is a priori, existing in us prior to experience, and Aquinas who seems to be caught between Augustine's platonic idealism and Aristotle's empiricism, though he is clear that beauty is not empirical knowledge.

Amongst contemporaries, Hans Urs von Balthasar was critical of those who tried to treat beauty as empirical and, in fact, of those who tried to make it subject to categories at all. He referred to it as a way of being rather than knowing. The concept of anamnesis is appropriately applied to his understanding of how it is that we perceive beauty. We could not appreciate beauty were God not to have given us that understanding.

Kant's moral analysis is problematic because his categorical imperatives, while attractive, have no foundation in his logic because they are founded only on the will rather than on the embodied nature of the human person. He is too dismissive of the reality of human experience. Though he and those who followed him were rejected by von Balthasar largely because they seek to categorize beauty as a kind of knowing rather than being, Kant and the empiricist philosopher David Hume, on the subject of beauty, are interesting because they apply a quite different logic to aesthetics than that which they apply to morals. They do want to assert that there is truth in beauty and to that extent we can agree with them and can use them to engage post-modernism.

The main finding that I want readers to take from this discussion of beauty is the connectedness of the transcendentals, so that the beauty of creation does have moral relevance and is a vital part of our relationship to God because of the connection that it establishes between us and the Creator. In its contemplation and in the way in which we treat the beauty of creation, we express our love for God as Creator. This will become clearer in the chapter on St Francis and others. The stewardship of creation goes far beyond us being merely responsible farmers, and mining and manufacturing sustainably.

St. Augustine is often quoted as saying:

> Does God proclaim Himself in the wonders of creation? No. All things proclaim Him, all things speak. Their beauty is the voice by which they announce God, by which they sing, "It is you who made me beautiful, not me myself but you".[183]

I want to stress the importance of natural beauty to theological reflection. When we admire a natural phenomenon such as a beautiful sunset it is possible to feel very close to the Creator,

---

[183] St Augustine, from his exposition on Psalm 148, retrieved from http://www.goodreads.com/quotes/show/34387 (accessed 10 January 2011).

whose mind has conjured up something so wonderful, despite us knowing the physics about how it has come to be- by the refraction of light through the atmosphere. Somehow the scientific explanation lacks something because the beauty has to be perceived to be appreciated. Not only has God created the sunset, he has created our capacity not just to see it but to see it in a particular way, which provokes that response in us which we associate with experiencing something beautiful.

When we hear a performance of a great piece of music, our thoughts turn to the composer whose ideas of order and harmony have given such meaning to the music. We can feel a great love for someone whom we have never met.

Writing as Cardinal Ratzinger, Pope Benedict XVI reflected:

> To admire the icons and the great masterpieces of Christian art in general, leads us on an inner way, a way of overcoming ourselves; thus in this purification of vision that is a purification of the heart, it reveals the beautiful to us, or at least a ray of it. In this way we are brought into contact with the power of the truth. I have often affirmed my conviction that the true apology of Christian faith, the most convincing demonstration of its truth against every denial, are the saints, and the beauty that the faith has generated. Today, for faith to grow, we must lead ourselves and the persons we meet to encounter the saints and to enter into contact with the Beautiful.[184]

A similar view has been expressed by Hans Urs von Balthasar. He indicates that apologetics should not be about arguing but about showing. He claims that rather than present someone with arguments for the existence of God, we are more likely to convince

---

184 Joseph Cardinal Ratzinger, *The Feeling of Things, the Contemplation of Beauty*, 2002, http://www.vatican.va/roman_curia/congregations/cfaith/documents/rc_con_cfaith_doc_20020824_ratzinger-cl-rimini_en.html (accessed 2010-2014)

them of his reality by showing them the beauty of revelation from the outset.[185] Whether he is right probably depends on the audience. There are many different paths to the faith.

Beauty is important to us. Beauty invokes a reaction in us and creates an interest. It is an experience of pleasure but is more than that - philosophers throughout the ages have expressed interest in the nature of our judgments about it and whether what is beautiful is a subjective judgment only or whether there is more to it. Philosophers have also tried to understand whether the experience of beauty has legitimacy both in the object itself and in the way in which it is perceived and understood. Is the sunset beautiful in itself? Is my perception and the response within me of appreciation of the sunset something that I learned – is it knowledge that I inherited or is it more than that, a way not of knowing but of being, of being one with my Creator in contemplation of His creation, at peace and in unity with Him?

When a person says something is beautiful he or she generally means more than that this observer finds it pleasurable. The observer expects others to also appreciate the object. There is something of an appeal to objectivity in a claim that something is beautiful. A statement claiming that it is beautiful is thus something that might be true or false.

Post-Humean views of beauty have tended to treat with derision any attempt to explain beauty objectively. There has been a kind of cultural puritanism which asserts that judgments about beauty are no more than expressions of pleasure and that to say that an artwork is good in an aesthetic sense, rather than being merely beneficial in a political or moral sense, is nonsense.

However some contemporary thinkers have persisted in devel-

---

[185] Hans Urs von Balthasar, *The Glory of the Lord: A Theological Aesthetics*, Vol 2, *Studies in Theological Style: Clerical Style*, trans. A. Louth et al, San Francisco, Ignatius Press, 1984, p. 166.

oping theories about beauty and the aesthetic. The philosopher Immanuel Kant has made a significant contribution to this discussion. He has pursued appreciation of beauty as a kind of knowing though others, such as Hans Urs von Balthasar as mentioned above, have insisted that is not a matter of knowing but being. In theology, there has been a growing interest in aesthetics often stimulated by the work of von Balthasar but also by the work of Paul Tillich, Emil Brunner, and Hans Küng; but theological interest in aesthetics is not new. It has had a strong role in the earliest Christian tradition. Notable contributors to the discussion have included Justin Martyr, Irenaeus, Origen, Dionysius and Augustine. Early in his scholarship, St Thomas Aquinas studied Dionysius and his aesthetics. For St Thomas, beauty is both transcendent and particular. It is attributable to both God and to things. It is attributable to things both sensible and supersensible. Daniel Gallagher also claims that insofar as it is a "transcendental" property, it is attributable to all things insofar as they exist because they are made by God.[186]

In this discussion about the importance of beauty in relation to the place of the environment in Theology, the following passage from von Balthasar makes an important claim:

> We no longer dare to believe in beauty and we make of it a mere appearance in order the more easily to dispose of it. Our situation today shows that beauty demands for itself at least as much courage and decision as do truth and goodness, and she will not allow herself to be separated and banned from her two sisters without taking them along with herself in an act of mysterious vengeance. We can be sure that whoever sneers at her name as if she were

---

[186] D.B. Gallagher, 'The Analogy of Beauty and the Limits of Theological Aesthetics', *Theandros*, vol. 3, no. 3, 2006, retrieved from http://www.theandros.com/beauty.html (accessed 29 December 2010).

the ornament of a bourgeois past – whether he admits it or not – can no longer pray and soon will no longer be able to love.[187]

Along similar lines he writes:

> ... Beauty is the last thing which the thinking intellect dares to approach, since only it dances as an uncontained splendour around the double constellation of the true and the good and their inseparable relation to one another. Beauty is the disinterested one, without which the ancient world refused to understand itself, a word which both imperceptibly and yet unmistakably has bid farewell to our new world, a world of interests, leaving it to its own avarice and sadness.[188]

7.3 Matters of Taste

When we say that a particular food or drink is pleasurable, we are simply reporting our own experience. Whether someone else will also find it pleasurable is simply a matter of taste. It is a subjective matter. At least up to a point, as there are some things that taste so awful that we could not imagine anyone finding them pleasurable. (The uniquely Australian appreciation of Vegemite might be a counterexample to that, though for most it does require a rather special context of hot buttered toast and the vegemite blending with the melted butter or margarine. I do not know anyone who eats it by the spoonful.)

However when we say that a work of art or a natural phenomenon is beautiful we are also saying that it is pleasurable, but it is a quite different meaning of pleasure and we do have an expectation that others will also find it pleasurable. Even a philosopher such as Kant

---

[187] Hans Urs von Balthasar, *The Glory of the Lord: A Theological Aesthetics, Vol 1 – Seeing the Form*, T&T Clark and Ignatius Press, 1982, p. 18.
[188] Ibid.

was able to recognize that beauty is not mere sensuous gratification, as in the pleasure of sensation, or of eating and drinking. Unlike such pleasures, pleasure in beauty is occasioned by the perceptual representation of a thing. It is also a disinterested form of pleasure. It is not related to any desire. It is not based on a desire nor does it give rise to a desire. In that sense pleasure in beauty is unlike pleasure in the agreeable, unlike pleasure in what is good for me, and unlike pleasure in what is morally good. According to Kant, all such pleasures are "interested" – they are bound up with desire. It may be that we have desires concerning beautiful things but so long as those desires are not intrinsic to the pleasure in beauty then the doctrine, that all pleasure is disinterested, is undisturbed.[189]

Kant asserts that the agreeable, the beautiful, and the good denote three different relations of representations to the feeling of pleasure and displeasure, a feeling in respect of which we distinguish different objects or modes of representation. Also, the corresponding expressions which indicate our satisfaction in them are different. The agreeable is what *gratifies* a man; the beautiful what simply *pleases* him; the good what is *esteemed* (approved) by him, that is, that on which he sets an objective worth.[190]

However to hold that a judgment that something is beautiful is to say that it is pleasurable does not quite capture the entire meaning. It is certainly a subjective judgment but it is more than that. The judgment that something is beautiful also has a normative element that Kant recognized. As Kant expressed it:

> ... when [someone] puts a thing on a pedestal and calls it beautiful, he demands the same delight from others. He judges not merely for himself, but for all men, and then speaks of beauty as if it were a property of things. Thus

---

189 'Aesthetic Judgement', *The Stanford Encyclopaedia of Philosophy*, 2003, http://plato.stanford.edu/entries/aesthetic-judgment/#1 (accessed 29 December 2010).
190 Kant, op. cit.

he says that the *thing* is beautiful; and it is not as if he counts on others agreeing with him in his judgment of liking owing to his having found them in such agreement on a number of occasions, but he *demands* this agreement of them. He blames them if they judge differently, and denies them taste, which he still requires of them as something they ought to have; and to this extent it is not open to men to say: Everyone has his own taste. This would be equivalent to saying that there is no such thing as taste, i.e. no aesthetic judgment capable of making a rightful claim upon the assent of all men.[191]

According to Kant the phrase "each to their own taste" only applies to judgments of niceness and nastiness, which Kant calls "judgments of agreeableness".[192] It may apply to food or wine, but it does not seem to be entirely appropriate when applied to a work of art or a natural phenomenon which we describe as beautiful. There is a sense in which a judgment that something is beautiful may be correct or incorrect.

A claim of this kind may provoke criticisms of intolerance and authoritarianism. But it is worth reflecting on the fact that the contemporary cultural insistence on relativism and subjectivity is itself intolerant and hypocritical. It is intolerant because what it means is that my subjective judgment is beyond criticism – I cannot be mistaken in my judgments. Second, it is hypocritical because in thus claiming that my judgment cannot be mistaken, I am asserting an authority for my judgments, the authority of infallibility. Only those who accept that there is a right and wrong in judgment can admit that they might be wrong in their judgment.[193]

The philosopher David Hume, who might be regarded as

---

191 Ibid.
192 Ibid.
193 'Aesthetic Judgement', *The Stanford Encyclopaedia of Philosophy*, op. cit.

the father of contemporary subjectivism, expressed this view succinctly: if you don't get pleasure from reading or listening to Shakespeare's *Sonnets*, we will think of you as being in error – not just your *judgment* but your *liking* is defective. Someone who thinks that there is "an equality of genius" between some inferior composer, on the one hand, and Bach, on the other, has a defective *sensibility*.[194] This stands in contrast to Hume's treatment of moral goodness.

The major point of interest in this philosophical discussion is its relevance the discussion about the beauty of creation. What judgment is being made by claiming that a wilderness, a beach, a mountain, a sunset, a tree, a species or a feature of a species is beautiful? What is the theological significance of so claiming?

7.4 Other Early Fathers and Beauty

St Justin lived in the 2nd century. He saw himself as a philosopher and used Platonic ideas to provide a philosophical defence of Christianity. For Plato the contemplation of forms, their structure and way of being, through true knowledge, is always something in which we can see the beautiful. All being is beautiful but is understood as a complex of differentiated ordered forms under the ever transcendental ultimate good. The idea of beauty is thus able to be related to God. Plato asserts that from an ascent of knowledge of sensuous beauty, in forms, in virtues, in various kinds of knowledge, one reaches knowledge of the beautiful. The ultimate uniquely beautiful is that which we desire to contemplate and with which we want to be connected because it is pure and touches truth and creates true virtue. Those who reach this level of contemplation deserve immortality and to be loved by the gods. St

---

[194] David Hume, 'Of the Standard of Taste', in E. Miller (ed.), *Essays: Moral, Political and Literary*, Indianapolis, Liberty, 1985, p. 230.

Justin relates this teaching of Plato to the person of Christ. Christ is the perfect image of God.[195]

For St Irenaeus, an immediate infinite God is present through the beauty and goodness of all His creation. Unity and universality are ruled by transcendent love. The unknowable God is knowable as universal intellect in His good economy, given for all creation.[196]

Origen of Alexandria, born 185 years after the birth of Jesus, is considered one of the greatest Christian theologians. He lived at a turbulent time in Christianity when there were conflicts between numbers of sects. Christianity was undergoing persecution by the central Roman government which was itself decadent and under attack from the barbarians. At that time Christian philosophy was not systematic and well developed. Trained in Greek philosophy, Origen set about applying the writing of Plato to Christianity and we owe a great debt to him for the clarity of his thinking and the development of consistent explanations for what had been revealed to us in Scripture and in the life, suffering and death of Christ.[197]

He is famous for composing the seminal work of Christian Neo-Platonism, his treatise *On First Principles*. Origen was the first truly philosophical thinker to turn his hand not only to a refutation of Gnosticism but to offer an alternative Christian system that was more rigorous and philosophically respectable than the mythological speculations of the various Gnostic sects.[198]

Nearly three hundred years after his death, Origen was con-

---

[195] G.E. Theissen (ed.), *Theological Aesthetics*, Grand Rapids, Eerdmans, 2006, pp. 10-11.
[196] E.F. Osborn, *Irenaeus of Lyons*, Cambridge and New York, Cambridge University Press, 2001, p. 51.
[197] 'Origen of Alexandria', *Internet Encyclopedia of Philosophy*, http://www.iep.utm.edu/origen-of-alexandria/ (accessed 29 December 2010).
[198] Ibid.

demned as a heretic by the Council of Constantinople which declared:

> If anyone does not anathematize Arius, Eunomius, Macedonius, Apollinaris, Nestorius, Eutyches and Origen, as well as their impious writings, as also all other heretics already condemned and anathematized by the Holy Catholic and Apostolic Church, and by the aforesaid four Holy Synods and [if anyone does not equally anathematize] all those who have held and hold or who in their impiety persist in holding to the end the same opinion as those heretics just mentioned: let him be anathema.[199]

This condemnation of Origen is sad really because he wrote speculatively at a time when many doctrines had not been defined. There seems to be something inherently unfair about condemning someone for heresy for speculation about matters that were not at that time declared doctrines. In other words, he made no conscious decision to be heretical but was seeking truth that had not been defined. The doctrine of the Trinity or of the creation of souls about which he formed views was not then a matter of doctrine. His errors were that he saw the Father as superior to the Son and the Son superior to the Holy Spirit rather than as participating equally in the one divine nature. He thought that our souls existed before conception and embraced dualism in that respect. He shared his dualism with St Augustine and that view was not corrected until the 13th century at the Council of Vienne which adopted the teaching of St Thomas Aquinas. In large part, the Church's difficulties with Origen seem to have involved some extreme views adopted by those describing themselves as his

---

[199] Paul Halsall, 'Fifth Ecumenical Council: Constantinople II, 553', *Medieval Sourcebook*, 1996, http://www.fordham.edu/halsall/basis/const2.html (accessed 29 December 2010).

followers, the Origenists. Their views were then retroactively attributed to Origen.[200]

Relevant to our discussion, Origen believed in the beauty of Jesus against claims at the time to his homeliness. The debate was over Isaiah 53.2:

> For he shot up right forth as a sapling,
> and as a root out of a dry ground;
> he had no form nor comeliness,
> that we should look upon him,
> nor beauty that we should delight in him.

And Psalm 45:

> 2 You are the most excellent (fairest) of men
> and your lips have been anointed with grace,
> since God has blessed you forever.
> 3 Gird your sword on your side, you mighty one;
> clothe yourself with splendor and majesty.

In relation to the beauty of creation, Origen starts from:

> ... the idea of an intimate relationship between God and the world and represents the latter as a necessary revelation of the former. It would be impious and absurd to maintain that there was a time when God did not show forth his essential attributes which make up his very being. He was never idle or quiescent. God's being is identical with his goodness and love, and his will is identical with his nature.[201]

Origen followed Plato who saw the world as imperfect, a copy

---

200 'Origen', *New World Encyclopedia*, http://www.newworldencyclopedia.org/entry/Origen#Impact (accessed 29 December 2010).
201 Philip Schaff, *History of the Christian Church, Volume II: Ante-Nicene Christianity. A.D. 100-325*, n. 969, retrieved from http://www.ccel.org/ccel/schaff/hcc2.txt (accessed 29 December 2010).

of a perfect rational eternal and changeless original. The beauty of a flower or a sunset, a piece of music or a love affair is an imperfect copy of Beauty itself. In this world of changing appearances, while you might catch a glimpse of that ravishing perfection, it will always fade. It's just a pointer to the perfect beauty of the eternal. Beauty is an example of a form, idea or universal. Many things can have the form or idea of beauty, but it exists only as an idea not in reality.[202]

For Plato, these Forms are perfect Ideals, but they are also more real than physical objects. The world of the Forms is rational and unchanging; the world of physical appearances is changeable and irrational, and only has reality to the extent that it succeeds in imitating the Forms. The mind or soul belongs to the Ideal world; the body and its passions are stuck in the muck of the physical world. So the best human life is one that strives to understand and to imitate the Forms as closely as possible: that life is the life of the mind, the life of the Philosopher (literally, the lover of wisdom).[203]

The divinity of Christ represented that absolute unchanging, eternal perfection of the Father but, as we have seen, Origen believed (heretically according to later dogma) that Christ was inferior because of the Incarnation and thus belonged to this inferior physical world. Creation originally reflected the perfect beauty of the Creator but has become affected by sin and hence contains only traces of that original beauty.[204]

Like Origen, Dionysius was a Neo-Platonist embracing Plato's idealism and adapting it to Christianity. Like Plato he understood Beauty as a transcendental along with Truth and Goodness. The

---

[202] D. Clowney, 'Plato's Aesthetics', *Aesthetics*, http://www.rowan.edu/open/philosop/clowney/Aesthetics/philos_artists_onart/plato.htm (accessed 29 December 2010).
[203] Ibid.
[204] Ronald E. Heine (trans.), *Origen: Homilies on Genesis and Exodus, Fathers of the Church*, vol. 71, Washington, Catholic University of America Press, 1982.

divine names "One", "Good" and "Being" are connected in Dionysian thought with the notions of "Life", "Wisdom" and "Light". The fundamental intuition of Dionysius is that the One is the beginning and the recapitulation of history. God, the One or Goodness Itself, is the "origin" of every other goodness. From the One, which is "eternally beautiful", "all things possess their existence, each kind being beautiful in its own manner". The One then is the "cause" of existence: "this One Good and Beautiful is in its Oneness the Cause of all the many beautiful and good things". All creation is thus linked to the Creator and all created things are therefore beautiful possessing their own order and harmony according to the divine plan.[205]

7.5 Aquinas

An intellectual giant in the Middle Ages was St Thomas Aquinas. In what is, in reality, an aside, St Thomas Aquinas famously claimed that beauty has three conditions and that a lack in any of these reduces beauty:

> For beauty includes three conditions, "integrity" or "perfection," since those things which are impaired are by the very fact ugly; due "proportion" or "harmony"; and lastly, "brightness" or "clarity," whence things are called beautiful which have a bright color.[206]

It is often said that beauty is in the eye of the beholder. This can be interpreted as saying that beauty is subjective and just a matter of taste. But the reflections of St Thomas and St Augustine provide a different perspective on what this saying might mean. For us, Beauty is an experience. Beauty has an impact upon us.

---

205 Constantine Scouteris, 'Platonic Elements in Pseudo-Dionysius Anti-Manichaean Ontology', http://www.orthodoxresearchinstitute.org/articles/dogmatics/scouteris_ontology.htm (accessed 2 January 2011).
206 Aquinas, *Summa Theologica I*, Q. 39, Art. 8, Obj. 5.

Something happens within the beholder when encountering beauty. Commenting on Dionysius, St Thomas writes:

> He shows how God is the Cause of brilliance, when he adds that God with a flash sends down to all creatures a share of His luminous ray, and it is the source of all light. These glittering communications of the divine ray should be understood according to the participation of likeness. And these communications are "pulchrifying," that is, producing beauty in things.[207]

Later St. Thomas, in the same commentary on Dionysius, writes:

> Brilliance pertains to the consideration of beauty ... Every form, by which a thing has being [*esse*], is a participation in the divine brilliance. This is why he [Dionysius] adds that 'individual things' are 'beautiful according to a character of their own,' that is, in accord with a proper form. Hence it is clear that the being [*esse*] of all things is derived from the divine Beauty.[208]

Referring to the passage from the *Summa*, quoted above, about the conditions of beauty, John Saward writes that the beautiful illuminates our *intellectus* with the intuition of understanding. The eyes and ears of our soul enable our vision to see the transcendent beauty present ontologically in all being.[209]

Sr. Thomas Mary McBride O.P. notes that St. Thomas, in his *Quaestiones Disputatae De Veritate*, distinguishes between the true and the good, and presents the insight that a spiritual substance

---

207 Aquinas, *Expositio in Dion. De div. Nom. 4.5-6*, as quoted in V.J. Bourke (trans.), *The Pocket Aquinas*, New York, Washington Square Press, 4th ed., 1965, pp. 269-270. cf. T.M. McBride, 'Beauty, Contemplation, and the Virgin Mary', http://www.christendom-awake.org/pages/mcbride/beauty.htm (accessed 5 January 2011).
208 Ibid., p. 272
209 John Saward, *The Beauty of Holiness and the Holiness of Beauty*, San Francisco, Ignatius Press, 1997, pp. 40-47.

relates to reality in two different ways. A human being directs himself at things by knowing them and desiring them. The object of knowledge is truth, while the object of desire is the good.[210]

McBride quotes St Thomas who argues that there is a way of relating to reality in which knowledge and desire are united in breathtaking vision:

> The splendor of truth and goodness radiating from the form captivates the one who *sees with love,* drawing him or her into a third way of ecstatic contemplation and intuitive wisdom. Beauty, therefore, is essentially a gift, a radiant vision presented to the eyes or ears of the beholder, a seeing or hearing of being clearly, that is, in the radiance of its inner splendor, *claritas.*[211]

Writing of the way in which beauty is received, St Thomas explains that we receive God's light differently depending on our intellect:

> ... the intellect which has more of the light of glory will see God the more perfectly; and he will have a fuller participation of the light of glory who has more charity; because where there is the greater charity, there is the more desire; and desire in a certain degree makes the one desiring apt and prepared to receive the object desired. Hence he who possesses the more charity, will see God the more perfectly, and will be the more beatified.[212]

McBride[213] understands ecstatic contemplation partaking of cognition as a *gift of wondrous seeing* with the eyes of the spirit. It is more than a knowing by which the known is in the knower,

---
210 T.M. McBride, 'Beauty, Contemplation, and the Virgin Mary', http://www.christendom-awake.org/pages/mcbride/beauty.htm (accessed 5 January 2011).
211 Aquinas, *Questiones Disputatae de Veritate*, Q. 21, Art. 3.
212 Aquinas, *Summa Theologica I*, Q. 12, Art. 6.
213 McBride, op. cit.

although it is that, but rather it is a being taken out of oneself by which *the knower is in the known*. She refers to von Balthasar's claim, "The light ... stems from the object which, while revealing itself to the subject, it draws the subject into the sphere of the object."[214]

McBride writes:

> ... beauty is therefore not so much an assimilation as being assimilated. Ecstasy resulting from beauty happens not by a movement toward the beautiful but rather by a dispositive attitude of receptivity in which one is inundated with love, peace and joy in the splendour of truth and goodness being revealed. Beauty is the gifted perfection of *seeing*. It unites the intellect and will in the innermost sanctuary of the soul.[215]

This way of understanding beauty focuses not on what makes something beautiful, but on how we perceive beauty, what quality of understanding we must possess in order to appreciate beauty.

On this issue, St Thomas writes:

> The beautiful is the same as the good, and they differ in aspect only. For since good is what all seek, the notion of good is that which calms the desire; while the notion of the beautiful is that which calms the desire, by being seen or known. Consequently those senses chiefly regard the beautiful, which are the most cognitive, viz. sight and hearing, as ministering to reason; for we speak of beautiful sights and beautiful sounds. But in reference to the other objects of the other senses, we do not use the expression "beautiful," for we do not speak of beautiful tastes, and beautiful odors. Thus it is evident that beauty adds to

---

214 Hans Urs von Balthasar, *The Glory of the Lord: A Theological Aesthetics*, Vol 1, op. cit., p. 181.
215 McBride, op. cit.

goodness a relation to the cognitive faculty: so that "good" means that which simply pleases the appetite; while the "beautiful" is something pleasant to apprehend.[216]

This leads McBride to claim that the proper place of beauty is in the spirit. The vision of beauty radiates and bears witness to the spiritual, awakening the most intimate depths of the human person. It captivates the mind and will in contemplative wonder and ecstatic contemplation. Beauty integrates the splendour of light with ecstatic joy. Ultimately, the vision of beauty bears witness to the divine beauty "which shines with dazzling light ... While remaining completely intangible and invisible, it fills minds that know how to close their eyes with the most beautiful splendours."[217]

Our interest in this subject is in natural beauty. What this analysis suggests is that the perception of beauty is something that happens in us so that the effect on us results from what it is that we receive, yet our ability to receive those effects is in part determined by us, by the actions of our intellectual soul. This suggests that we could be blind to beauty if we are inadequately developed.

7.6 The Relationship of Truth, Goodness and Beauty

The relationship between the transcendentals has a bearing on this. Might we, for instance, describe a depiction of great evil as beautiful? Would we describe something as beautiful that was misleading? In both cases the evil or the deception would have severed the connection between what is beautiful and the divine.

Some time ago I visited the National Gallery of Victoria in Melbourne. There was a work of great execution and realism

---

216 Aquinas, *Summa Theologica I:II*, Q. 27, Art. 1
217 Dionysius the Areopagite, *Theologia Mystica*, as quoted by Pope John Paul II, 'General Audience', *L'Osservatore Romano*, 26 January 2000, p. 11 (cf. McBride, op. cit.).

showing several people all of whom were nude and engaged in a variety of sexual liaisons of varying depravity. The painting made me pause for a moment to wonder whether I was too much of a prude to appreciate what I found confronting. I have often appreciated works depicting nudity so that was not the issue. Then it struck me that despite the skill in the work, the order and symmetry of the bodies, the beauty of the human form being skilfully depicted, the subject matter rendered it not a beautiful work. The picture did not affect me the way in which truly beautiful works had such as two Dutch favourites of mine: Rembrandt's *Two Old Men Disputing* (which I imagine to be Peter and Paul) and Nicholas Maes' *Old Woman at Prayer* both of which, despite the constant familiarity of prints of them on my office wall, never fail to affect me. Part of what makes a great work of art is the light of goodness and truth, the meaning that shines from it. The light shining from the scene of depravity was not light at all.

A picture that takes my interest is the Jean Paul David depiction of the *Assassination of Marat in his Bath*. It is in many ways a remarkable picture because of the use of light and colour and the story it tells. However, to my way of thinking, it is not a beautiful painting, despite its being worth a fortune and despite the painter's intention of depicting Marat as a martyr of the revolution. Somehow the wickedness of Marat and the despair of his assailant render the painter's intent, in relation to depicting his friend's death, false, and the painting thus not beautiful. Had there been a different story behind the painting it might have been considered beautiful. The many depictions of the deaths of true martyrs seem somehow to be different in their effects from this. I was struck, similarly, by the change wrought in recent times to the public appreciation of the music and art of Rolf Harris after his conviction for sex crimes against children. We do connect the transcendentals.

7.7 Natural Beauty

I began this account of beauty referring to our ability to appreciate the beauty of a sunset or a rainbow, a forest or a mountainside, the breathtaking sights to be seen on a coral reef, or a condor in flight, a lion or an elephant in natural habitat. The question of what makes such phenomena beautiful is both a question about what makes them beautiful and about what make us perceive beauty. The first is a question about the world around us. The second is a question about ourselves. In relation to the latter, what we see as beautiful may not be unrelated to the other transcendentals. Whether something is beautiful can be affected by the meaning we attach to it.

This suggests that our appreciation of a work of art will, to some extent, depend on what we take to be in the mind of the artist. The work expresses the meaning given to it by the artist. I thus find it completely puzzling that, with some contemporary works of art, the artists choose not to give a name or a meaning. There was for a time a public work of art on display in Melbourne in the civic square that is now known as Federation Square. Initially the artist, Ron Robertson-Swann, gave it no name so the public called it the "Yellow Peril". It is built of large thick flat sheets of prefabricated steel painted yellow. Later, when a name was demanded, the artist called it, vaguely and ambiguously, "Vaults" though the shape was said to display movement. After much ridicule it was relocated to the mud flats of Batman Park beside the river where few could see it and where it was neglected. More recently it was renovated and given a home at the Centre for Contemporary Art.[218]

In the first instance what frustrated me mostly was the absence of a name and meaning from the artist. I was prepared to be open

---

218 Alan Attwood, 'Peril in the Square: The Sculpture that Challenged a City', *The Age*, 19 June 2004, http://www.theage.com.au/articles/2004/06/16/1087244973120. html?from=storyrhs (accessed 2010-2014).

to what it meant but on neither finding meaning in its appearance nor being given a meaning by the artist I could not appreciate it, and I suspect that I was not alone. The Melbourne public might have been more tolerant if we had been told the artist's intent. I could not regard it as beautiful without attribution of meaning. The "Yellow Peril" ended up being cast out of the square and left to rot.

On the other hand we readily appreciate the beauty of natural phenomena without a sign or any other communication to tell us what a phenomenon means. The sunset simply is a beautiful sunset, the mountain is a beautiful mountain, and the lion is a beautiful beast. Is that because they are natural phenomena and we see them as works of God's graciousness and goodness? Is it because God has created in us an appreciation of creation? I have never heard someone describe a sunset as ugly. Even a sunset amongst angry storm clouds, and perhaps the fear of an approaching fierce storm, is still beautiful.

What the saints have seen in the various natural phenomena of creation is the beauty of the Creator. The Creator's beauty, truth and goodness communicate to and are communicated by the beauty of divine creation. Despite scientific explanations of how those phenomena came to be, they retain the beauty of the Creator and they tell us of His divine nature in much the same way that a work of art or a musical composition says something to us of the artist or composer.

7.8 Stewardship and Beauty

The point of this analysis has been to attempt to explain why it is that a Christian perspective of the environment, in terms of dominion and stewardship, is not utilitarian and not anthropocentric. The beauty of the environment speaks to us of the Creator and in its contemplation we are in relationship with the Creator. For believers, it is not enough that we think in terms of sustainability and of "managing" the environment as a set of resources, our stewardship is also concerned not only about our impact on the beauty of God's creation but also about our relationship to God, expressed in our relationship to His Creation, such that our contemplation of the environment becomes an expression of our love for the Creator. We will return to this topic when we discuss St Francis of Assisi.

The experience of natural beauty is a puzzle for us. It is an important part of the experience of God and as such it is part of our being. It is also a kind of knowing and that is the way in which Augustine and Thomas saw it and they thought it was worth exploring to try to identify the elements of that knowledge and its relationship to the other transcendentals. It is significant that we do not hold that something which expresses a falsehood or a moral depravity can be beautiful. Essential to the beauty of a sunset is that it is God's creation and we stand before it in awe despite knowing the physics of refraction that produces it. Importantly creation differs from even the best of man-made art because of the nature of the Creator and the expression of that nature in His Creation.

In that respect, I think that what von Balthasar has claimed about *showing* rather than *arguing* the truth is important even though I do not think that therefore there is no place for arguing the truth. There is a place for St Paul in evangelism. It is not enough that Jesus lived amongst and died for us, we still need to explore what the Jesus event means as well as appreciating the beauty of His incarnated holiness. There are many pathways to the faith. For some, the beauty of the Word, of the Christ event, of all God's creation and of religious art, religious architecture, and religious liturgy will be dominant in what brings conviction and commitment.

So the place that natural beauty has in our lives comes to us through it being an expression of the mind of the Creator and in our being close to it: in immersing ourselves in contemplation of His creation we find ourselves to be one with the Creator. This contemplation, for a mind that is receptive to it, brings about an extraordinary sense of peace and fulfilment because it expresses not just His beauty but also His truth and goodness.

We are stewards, as Pope John Paul II acknowledged when he demanded that: "States must increasingly share responsibility, in complementary ways, for the promotion of a natural and social environment that is both peaceful and healthy."[219] The Pope claimed further that:

> Theology, philosophy and science all speak of a harmonious universe, of a "cosmos" endowed with its own integrity, its own internal, dynamic balance. *This order must be respected.* The human race is called to explore this order, to examine it with due care and to make use of it while safeguarding its integrity.[220]

The International Theological Commission addressed the issues of communion and stewardship:

> Human beings, created in the image of God, are persons called to enjoy communion and to exercise stewardship in a physical universe. The activities entailed by interpersonal communion and responsible stewardship engage the spiritual - intellectual and affective – capacities of human persons, but they do not leave the body behind. Human beings are physical beings sharing a world with other physical beings. Implicit in the Catholic theology of the imago Dei is the profound truth that the material world creates the conditions for the engagement of human persons with one another.[221]

---

[219] Pope John Paul II, *Peace with God the Creator, Peace with all Creation*, op. cit.
[220] Ibid.
[221] International Theological Commission, op. cit., n. 26.

Our relationship with the environment is one of stewardship and with that stewardship comes the need to protect the sustainability of the resources that the created order provides for us. But the relationship is more than that. The created order is a system in ecological balance and we can affect that balance. In trying to understand that order we need to seek to understand the mind of the Creator and, in seeing His thought expressed in His creation, to seek a communion with that nature and through it with Him. Clearly thinking along these lines, the Commission wrote:

> The Christian theology of creation contributes directly to the resolution of the ecological crisis by affirming the fundamental truth that visible creation is itself a divine gift, the "original gift," that establishes a "space" of personal communion. Indeed, we could say that a properly Christian theology of ecology is an application of the theology of creation ... Given that the inner life of the Blessed Trinity is one of communion, the divine act of creation is the gratuitous production of partners to share in this communion. In this sense, one can say that the divine communion now finds itself "housed" in the created cosmos. For this reason, we can speak of the cosmos as a place of personal communion.[222]

In his 2010 World Day of Peace message, Pope Benedict XVI declared, *"If you want to cultivate peace, protect creation."* He explained that the quest for peace would become easier if all were to acknowledge the indivisible relationship between God, human beings and the whole of creation. He spoke of the special role for Christians in contemplating the cosmos and its marvels in light of the creative work of the Father and the redemptive work of

---
222 Ibid., n. 74

Christ, who by his death and resurrection has reconciled to God "all things, whether on earth or in heaven" (Col 1:20).[223]

> Protecting the natural environment in order to build a world of peace is ... a duty incumbent upon each and all. It is an urgent challenge, one to be faced with renewed and concerted commitment; it is also a providential opportunity to hand down to coming generations the prospect of a better future for all. May this be clear to world leaders and to those at every level who are concerned for the future of humanity: the protection of creation and peacemaking are profoundly linked![224]

The theology of the beauty of all creation is not separable from our understanding of deification or divination, understood as our union with God, and the role of divine grace. The capacity to perceive beauty in the beautiful and to be affected by it is a grace that brings us closer to God. It seems also to give us some sense of what communion with God, which is our ultimate end, may be. When we stand in awe of the beauty of a natural phenomenon, as believers we may feel a sense of being in God's presence. There is a parallel in our appreciation of what we understand to be the mind of an artist who communicates with us by arresting meaning through the work. A great piece of music or a great painting or sculpture can have a profound effect on us and that effect makes us conscious of the artist. Of course all human creations are marred by sin, as is our perception of them. How much richer is the potential impact on us of a beautiful natural phenomenon because of its authorship, causing us to wonder about the Creator, as much as about the beauty of the phenomenon itself? That wonder is enhanced by the science that explains not just the complexity of the phenomenon but also the complexity of the process by which

---

223 Pope Benedict XVI, *If You Want to Cultivate Peace, Protect Creation*, op. cit., n. 12.
224 Ibid.

the phenomenon came to be and by our own sense of the mystery of the way in which we have the capacity to appreciate its beauty. It seems that God's design not only produced great beauty but also our capacity to appreciate it. This seems to have a relationship to our own deification in coming to closer union with the Creator through the experience of beauty in natural phenomena. The latter reflects both our own deification and the deification of all creation. One of the most interesting aspects of deification is whether the Incarnation was always to be part of creation or whether it was a divine response necessitated by sin in order to redeem us and restore our capacity for union with God.[225]

---

225 Adam G. Cooper, *Naturally Human, Supernaturally God: Deification in Preconciliar Catholicism*, US, Fortress Press, 2014.

8

THE SACRAMENTALITY OF CREATION: THE INVISIBLE IN THE VISIBLE

8.1 Sacraments and Sacramentality

For Catholics the word "sacrament" has a particular meaning referring to the seven sacraments instituted by Christ: Baptism, Penance, Communion, Confirmation, Marriage, Holy Orders and the Sacrament of the Sick. They have in common the fact that they are efficacious signs of grace, instituted by Christ and entrusted to the Church, by which divine life is dispensed to us.[226]

The term "sacrament" has a wider usage within the Church, however. The Second Vatican Council referred to the Church itself as a sacrament:

> ... the Church, in Christ, is a sacrament – a sign and instrument, that is of communion, with God and of the unity of the entire human race ...[227]

> Christ when he was lifted up from the earth drew all humanity to himself. Rising from the dead he sent his life-giving Spirit upon his disciples and through him set up his body which is the church as the universal sacrament of salvation.[228]

St Augustine used the word "sacramentum" widely to mean anything that is a sacred sign to be received in a holy fashion

---

[226] *Catechism of the Catholic Church*, n. 1131.
[227] Second Vatican Council, *Lumen Gentium*, n. 1.
[228] Ibid., n. 48.

because it carries the mind to a transcendent reality.[229] Of creation he writes:

> For, though the voices of the prophets were silent, the world itself, by its well-ordered changes and movements, and by the fair appearance of all visible things, bears a testimony of its own, both that it has been created, and also that it could not have been created save by God, whose greatness and beauty are unutterable and invisible.[230]

8.2 The Early Fathers and Creation as Witness to the Creator

The Early Fathers also reflected on all creation as a sign and an instrument of God as Creator and of His presence amongst us. St Basil the Great wrote:

> I want creation to penetrate you with so much admiration that wherever you go, the least plant may bring you the clear remembrance of the Creator ... One blade of grass or one speck of dust is enough to occupy your entire mind in beholding the art with which it has been made ... The earth is the Lord's and the fullness thereof. O God, enlarge within us the sense of fellowship with all living things, even our brothers, the animals, to whom Thou gavest the earth as their home in common with us ... We remember with shame that in the past we have exercised the high dominion of man with ruthless cruelty so that the voice of the earth, which should have gone up to thee in song, has been a groan of pain. May we realize that they live, not for us alone, but for themselves and for Thee and that they love the sweetness of life.[231]

---

[229] St Augustine, *City of God*, bk. 10, chapter 5.
[230] St Augustine, *City of God*, bk. 11, chapter 4.
[231] St Basil the Great (329-379), Hexaemeron (Homily V): 'The Germination of the Earth', in O. Davies (ed.), *Gateway to Paradise / Basil the Great*, trans. T. Witherow, Brooklyn, New City Press, 1991.

St Augustine often referred to the beauty of creation as a sacrament and appealed to us in the following way:

> Some people read books in order to find God. Yet there is a great book, the very appearance of created things. Look above you; look below you! Note it; read it! God, whom you wish to find, never wrote that book with ink. Instead, He set before your eyes the things that He had made. Can you ask for a louder voice than that?[232]

St. John of Damascus said something similar:

> The whole earth is a living icon of the face of God ... I do not worship matter. I worship the Creator of matter who became matter for my sake, who willed to take His abode in matter, who worked out my salvation through matter. Never will I cease honoring the matter which wrought my salvation! I honor it, but not as God. Because of this I salute all remaining matter with reverence, because God has filled it with his grace and power. Through it my salvation has come to me.[233]

As did St. Bernard of Clairvaux:

> Believe an expert: you will find something far greater in the woods than in books. Trees and stones will teach you that which you cannot learn from the masters.[234]

And St John Chrysostom added so eloquently:

> Nature is Our Best Teacher
> From the creation,

---

[232] St Augustine, Sermon, Mai 126.6, as cited in V.J. Bourke (trans.), *The Essential Augustine*, Indianapolis, Hackett Publishing, 1974, p. 123.

[233] St John of Damascus, *Writings/Saint John of Damascus, The Fathers of the Church: A New Translation*, vol. 37, trans. F.H. Chase Jr., Washington, Catholic University of America Press, 1970.

[234] St Bernard of Clairvaux, Epistola CVI, sect. 2, in E. Churton (trans.), *The Early English Church*, London, Burns, 1840, p. 324.

learn to admire the Lord!
And if any of the things which you
see exceed your comprehension,
and you are not able to find the reason for its existence,
then for this reason,
glorify the Creator that the wisdom of His works
surpasses your own understanding.
Indeed the magnitude and beauty of creation
and also the very manner of it,
display a God Who is the artificer of the universe.
He has made the mode of this creation to be our best teacher, compounding all things in a manner that transcends the course of nature.[235]

8.3 Humanity as Witness to God

Under the heading of "sacramentality" there is the idea that in our observation of the creation around us and in us we can witness the divine nature imprinted, as it were, on creation. We understand this in ourselves through the *imago Dei* that in the beginning, before the effects of sin, humanity was formed in the image and likeness of God. Part of humanity's likeness to God is that we can think, reason, make decisions, plan, doubt, love, affirm and wonder, all those capacities that are needed for us to be like God, as lovers. Importantly we are capable of both good and evil and have the freedom to choose them. The capacity to do that is not just a freedom, but requires an ability to be aware of ourselves. We could not sin unless we had a concept of our being different by having acted differently. In some ways life would be easier if we

---

235 St John Chrysostom, 'Homily 12 on the Statutes', in W.R.W. Stephens (trans.), *Nicene and Post-Nicene Fathers*, First Series, vol. 9, ed. P. Schaff, Buffalo, Christian Literature Publishing, 1889, retrieved from http://www.newadvent.org/fathers/190112.htm (accessed 2010-2014).

were automatons acting out in imitation of God's goodness, but without free will and rationality we would be much less like God, because we would lack the capacity for love and for friendship. Love involves a concept of self and a concept of another and of the relationship between the two and how one is able to form and develop that relationship as a completely free act. Love is a decision through which we witness to God's love.

In this respect we are different to animals. Animals lack the freedom that we have: our freedom comes through our self-awareness that allows us to shape our own characters. Preceding the capacity to sin is, first and foremost, the capacity to identify the good and to seek the good by freely chosen actions. St Thomas Aquinas acknowledges that animals differ from us in that they lack the coalition of ideas which he calls the cogitative power. He discusses the capacity that animals have to perceive something which is not immediately available to the senses, such as a bird gathering straws in order to build a nest. The concept of a nest is an idea that is not immediately apparent to the senses, but the bird in gathering the straw clearly does so in order to build the nest. Bower birds are most interesting in that the male will go to extraordinary lengths to beautify the nest using whatever it is that may be at hand to make the nest attractive, not just functional. When they go out foraging for material for the beautification of the nest do they do so instinctively or do they do so with an abstract idea of the nest in mind? Aquinas seeks to distinguish between humans and animals in the following way:

> Now, we must observe that as to sensible forms there is no difference between man and other animals; for they are some similarly immuted by the extrinsic sensible. But there is a difference as to the above intentions: for other animals perceive these intentions only by some natural instinct, while man perceives them by means of coalition

of ideas. Therefore the power by which in other animals is called the natural estimative, in man is called the "cogitative", which by some sort of collation discovers these intentions.[236]

Aquinas also points to the function of imagination in humans so that we may take a concept such as goldness and a concept such as a mountain and imagine a gold mountain without ever having seen such a thing. He would argue that the bower bird is acting instinctively when it collects a bright or differently shaped object and takes it back to the nest rather than that the bird has an idea of the completed nest in mind and imagines how it might look with the addition of the acquired objects. What is significant for our discussion of evolution is that Aquinas argues that the intellect is a power of the soul. Popes Benedict XVI and John Paul II accept evolution of the body but not of the soul. This would seem to imply that the specific likeness to God in our intellectual capacity, and spiritual life particularly, is a result not of the evolution of the body but of the divine creation of a specific individual human soul. We will talk more about this later.

8.4 Trinitarian Anthropology

Seeing ourselves as sacramental makes sense particularly with reference to our capacity to love. We can see that in giving oneself in religious life or in marriage one is seeking to give witness to God's love. One seeks to make of oneself a complete gift of oneself. The giving imitates God's giving, as Creator, as Christ on the Cross, as a person of the Holy Trinity. The marriage analogy to the relationship between the persons of the Trinity is something of a novelty of recent times, particularly in the encyclical *Mulieris Dignitatem* and in the John Paul II papal catechesis on the theology of the body. This is often called "Trinitarian anthropology".

---

236 Aquinas, *Summa Theologica I*, Q. 78, Art. 4.

The marriage analogy applies to Christ and the Church (Eph 5:23, John 3:27-30, 2 Cor 11:2, Rev 21:2 & 9) and our likeness to God is expressed in Genesis (Gen 1: 26–27, 5: 1–3, 9:1–7). In recent times, on the basis of marriage being a witness to Christ's love for the Church and of men and women being *imago Dei*, Pope John Paul II developed a Trinitarian anthropology in which he claims that the love between man and woman is a witness to the love of the Triune God, the love between the persons of the Holy Trinity. Pope John Paul II expresses the witness of marriage in the following way in *Mulieris Dignitatem n. 7*:

> The fact that man "created as man and woman" is the image of God means not only that each of them individually is like God, as a rational and free being. It also means that man and woman, created as a "unity of the two" in their common humanity, are called to live in a communion of love, and in this way to mirror in the world the communion of love that is in God, through which the Three Persons love each other in the intimate mystery of the one divine life. The Father, Son and Holy Spirit, one God through the unity of the divinity, exist as persons through the inscrutable divine relationship. Only in this way can we understand the truth that God in himself is love (cf. 1 *Jn* 4:16).

The analogy of the relationship between the spouses in marriage and the persons of the Holy Trinity is a very rich analogy. However it is an analogy that has been controversial in the Church. St. Augustine rebukes those who seek to discover the divine image of the Trinity in a trinity of persons which belong to the natural human order: an image which would be realized in marriage by the presence of man, woman and child.[237] The notion that he takes to task is the view:

---

237 St Augustine, *De Trinitate*, bk. 12, chapter 5, http://www.newadvent.org/fathers/130112.htm (accessed 2010-2014).

> ... that a trinity of the image of God in three persons, so far as regards human nature, can so be discovered as to be completed in the marriage of male and female and in their offspring; in that the man himself, as it were, indicates the person of the Father, but that which has so proceeded from him as to be born, that of the Son; and so the third person as of the Spirit, is, they say, the woman, who has so proceeded from the man as not herself to be either son or daughter, although it was by her conception that the offspring was born.[238]

St Augustine attacks this on several grounds but the principal one is that in Genesis man and woman are both made equally in the image and likeness of God, who is three persons, and neither is particularly in the likeness of one person or another of the Trinity. This is quite different from the analogy that Pope John Paul II drew between the communion of persons in marriage and the communion of the persons of the Trinity. In the pope's thought there is no analogy between the man or the woman and any particular person of the Trinity. The Genesis text is quite clear in saying that both man and woman were created in the divine image. In the light of the New Testament we know that to mean that they were created in the image of the triune God. St Augustine seems to be silent on this matter of the marital love of a man and a woman being a witness to the triune God in the sense that their communion is a witness to the communion between the persons of the Holy Trinity.

8.5 All Creation

Seeing ourselves as sacramental is possible because we believe that we are made in the image and likeness of God. The Fathers, however, also saw all creation as manifesting the Creator. St.

---

238 Ibid.

Augustine takes the statement "and God saw that it was good" (Genesis 1) and considers what "good" in this sense could mean:

> The assertion of the goodness of the created work follows the act of creation in order to emphasize that the work corresponded with the goodness that was the reason for its creation. Now if this goodness is rightly interpreted as the Holy Spirit, then the whole united Trinity is revealed to us in its works.[239]

The puzzle for us is to understand how we can apply divine goodness to all creation. It is one thing to marvel at the mountains and the seas, the sunsets and the sunrises, and the beauty of so many of God's creatures. However the lion devours the gazelle. When the mountain began it probably caused death and destruction through lava flows, earthquakes and tsunami. Why make the influenza virus or HIV? Yet at the same time who can watch a David Attenborough documentary and not marvel at the intricacy of a bird dancing, or preparing a bower, to attract a mate? Apparent in nature is not only its immense complexity, but also its relatedness. A scientist who sees under a microscope the characteristic weal of the astigmatid mite, that can so devastate a flock of sheep, might find it hard to comprehend how such a creature could be considered to display divine goodness. Nevertheless, like us, it is part of divine creation, this immense ecology in which every small item has its place.

Somewhere between the Early Fathers and the industrial and technological marvels of our own time our culture lost much of its sense of reverence and awe for the divine and for divine creation. Through science and the enlightenment we thought that we could master our environment and we surrounded ourselves with man-made items in which to seek comfort. Western culture also stopped seeing the environment and ourselves as having a

---

239 St Augustine, *City of God*, bk. 11, chapter 24.

teleology, a purpose. This permitted us to see the environment as an exploitable resource. Even now, when we have realised that many resources are finite and not renewable, we find it difficult to find a paradigm to apply to this new challenge of finding alternatives to our consumption of resources.

It is worth reflecting on pre-industrial theology and the different way in which the Early Fathers saw the world. They envisaged a world in which God is an active presence. Every creature is the result of an independent act of creation. This creation has a hierarchy in which humans are at the top, their intelligence making them, of all creation, most like the divine nature. However the Fathers saw each creature, not just humans, manifesting something of that divine nature.

Darwinism and the industrial and technological revolution had a dramatic effect on the enlightenment. Nature ceased to have a teleology. It was, after all, the result of accidents and natural selection. Even many theists stopped imagining that God played an active role. As Jame Schaefer expresses it, "... the world was like a clock that God created, wound up and left to unwind on its own without any interference, interaction or adjustment."[240]

Interestingly Darwinism and contemporary science support a notion of a world as a vast ecology, emergent, evolutionary, dynamic, unpredictable and holistic.[241] If there is one thing that is clear from the current debate over climate, carbon and global warming, it is that we have a very limited capacity to understand the causes of events and to predict future outcomes. Who can say where or when the next cyclone or tsunami may cause devastation?

The science of forecasting anything is the application of a model that explains current events on the assumption that if it has

---

240 Jame Schaefer, *Theological Foundations for Environmental Ethics*, Georgetown University Press, 2009, p. 81.
241 Ibid.

been sufficiently tried and found accurate it may be reliable for future events extrapolated from current data. But often there are multiple models to be applied which have had success applied to past events, but which produce a range of differing outcomes about future events. That is why prediction of climate change is such a matter of dispute. Science has its limitations.

Importantly, science is also showing us that we are so dependent on air, land and water and that what we do with them can affect not just this generation but those to come.

8.6 Two Different Ideas of Evolution

It is important to separate two different versions of evolution: the version of the likes of Richard Dawkins, Christopher Hitchens or Stephen Hawking who have it that the universe evolved simply as a matter of chance and natural selection, and the version implied by Pope John Paul II and accepted by Pope Benedict XVI who have it that the universe is created, is sustained by God and evolves according to His plan and natural laws for it, but does not include the evolution of the human soul which is individually created by God. The latter version is inconsistent with fundamentalist theories of evolution, such as those held by Dawkins, Hawking and Hitchens, who understand that resulting from a Big Bang there was just matter, that that matter evolved to form life and that life subsequently emerged as animal then human, and that all that was a result of chance, change and the effect of natural selection. Note, as discussed earlier, that fundamentalist evolutionary theory presupposes no creator and there is no room for purpose or design in that account. It is not the evolutionary theory of Charles Darwin who still believed the Creator is the origin of all creation and of the marvels of evolution.

Some find it difficult to accept evolution because it means that human beings came from animals: at some point an animal became human. However the biblical account is even worse. Genesis tells us that God made us by forming us from dust: "... then the Lord God formed man of dust from the ground, and breathed into his nostrils the breath of life, and man became a living being ..." (Genesis 2:7).

It is a small step from understanding that we evolved from mere matter, to vegetable, to animal life, and then to human life, to relating this account to the Genesis account of creation – God giving form to matter and then breathing a human soul into that form – to understanding that, having evolved to a point, via an evolutionary process of God's design, God then considered the form that we had reached to be suitable to receive a human intellectual and immortal soul. Science shows us much about the molecules that form a human embryo and then develop to be a rational adult person. However, the study of the molecules that form the human body does not yet reveal the function of our intellectual processes, though it may well do so in the future. However, our reasons for behaving as we do are not entirely subject to biological determinism. As lovers we have free will, a free will itself informed by science, and part of the mystery of being a human being is that we adapt to the information we receive and are conscious of being able to choose. The teaching of the Church, as defined by Pope John Paul II, would seem to require that the mystery of those intellectual capacities that human beings possess, that make us so distinctively the image of God, are not the result of evolution but are the result of the individual creation by God of our immortal souls.[242] This seems to be a major point of difference between fundamentalist evolutionists and compatibilists.

As Cardinal Newman expressed it:

> As to the Divine Design, is it not an instance of incomprehensibly and infinitely marvellous Wisdom and Design to

---

[242] Pope John Paul II, *Truth Cannot Contradict Truth*, op. cit.

have given certain laws to matter millions of ages ago, which have surely and precisely worked out, in the long course of those ages, those effects which He from the first proposed. Mr. Darwin's theory need not then to be atheistical, be it true or not; it may simply be suggesting a larger idea of Divine Prescience and Skill. Perhaps your friend has got a surer clue to guide him than I have, who have never studied the question, and I do not [see] that 'the accidental evolution of organic beings' is inconsistent with divine design – It is accidental to us, not to God.[243]

What is central to our faith is that we are God's creation. Pope John Paul II claimed that the human soul is individually created by God.[244] In his account of Genesis, Pope Benedict XVI expressed it in the following way:

> Human life stands under God's special protection, because each human being, however wretched or exalted he or she may be, however sick or suffering, however good-for-nothing or important, whether born or unborn, whether incurably ill or radiant with health – each one bears God's breath in himself or herself, each one is God's image. This is the deepest reason for the inviolability of human dignity, and upon it is founded ultimately every civilization. When the human person is no longer seen as standing under God's protection and bearing God's breath, then the human being begins to be viewed in utilitarian fashion. It is then that the barbarity appears that tramples upon human dignity. And vice versa: When this is seen, then a high degree of spirituality and morality is plainly evident.[245]

On the matter of evolution he said:

---

243 Newman, *The Letters*, op. cit.
244 Pope John Paul II, *Truth Cannot Contradict Truth*, op. cit.
245 Ratzinger, *'In the beginning ... '*, op. cit.

> Currently, I see in Germany, but also in the United States, a somewhat fierce debate raging between so-called "creationism" and evolutionism, presented as though they were mutually exclusive alternatives: those who believe in the Creator would not be able to conceive of evolution, and those who instead support evolution would have to exclude God. This antithesis is absurd because, on the one hand, there are so many scientific proofs in favour of evolution which appears to be a reality we can see and which enriches our knowledge of life and being as such. But on the other, the doctrine of evolution does not answer every query, especially the great philosophical question: where does everything come from? And how did everything start which ultimately led to man?[246]

In the account of evolution accepted by the Catholic Church is the certainty that the universe is created by God out of nothing and that the human soul is individually created. There is then a close link between humanity and the rest of creation. We are part of creation and our genome indicates that common history with the animals. This view of our proximity to animals is not a new view.

Aquinas was no believer in evolution, in fact he would seem to have been opposed, at all, to the idea of animals (including man as a rational animal) coming to be from a seed. He seems to have believed in spontaneous generation.

> Since the generation of one thing is the corruption of another, it was not incompatible with the first formation of things, that from the corruption of the less perfect the more perfect should be generated. Hence animals

---

246 Pope Benedict XVI, *Meeting of the Holy Father Benedict XVI with the Clergy of the Dioceses of Belluno-Feltre and Treviso*, 24 July 2007, http://www.vatican.va/holy_father/benedict_xvi/speeches/2007/july/documents/hf_ben-xvi_spe_20070724_clero-cadore_en.html (accessed 2010-2014).

generated from the corruption of inanimate things, or of plants, may have been generated then.[247]

However he does seem to have an idea of mutation and possibly natural selection, though the latter might be stretching his understanding.

> The same thing is true of those substances which Empedocles said were produced at the beginning of the world, such as the 'ox-progeny', i.e., half ox and half man. For if such things were not able to arrive at some end and final state of nature so that they would be preserved in existence, this was not because nature did not intend this [a final state], but because they were not capable of being preserved. For they were not generated according to nature, but by the corruption of some natural principle, as it now also happens that some monstrous offspring are generated because of the corruption of seed.[248]

Aquinas also seems to be generally puzzled by questions such as how the first animals could have come to be because they could not have come from putrefaction. A similar question arises for us in relation to trying to reconcile the creation of humans and animals if there was no death before the Fall. Aquinas addresses the idea that some species came into existence after the seventh day by saying:

> Nothing entirely new was afterwards made by God, but all things subsequently made had in a sense been made before in the work of the six days. Some things, indeed, had a previous experience materially, as the rib from the side of Adam out of which God formed Eve; whilst others

---

247 Aquinas, *Summa Theologica I*, Q. 72, Art. 1.
248 Aquinas, *Commentary on Aristotle's Physics: Book II*, Lectio 14 (199 a 34-b 33), n. 263, retrieved from http://dhspriory.org/thomas/Physics2.htm#14 (accessed 2010-2014).

existed not only in matter but also in their causes, as those individual creatures that are now generated existed in the first of their kind. Species, also, that are new, if any such appear, existed beforehand in various active powers; so that animals, and perhaps even new species of animals, are produced by putrefaction by the power which the stars and elements received at the beginning. Again, animals of new kinds arise occasionally from the connection of individuals belonging to different species, as the mule is the offspring of an ass and a mare; but even these existed previously in their causes, in the works of the six days. Some also existed beforehand by way of similitude, as the souls now created. And the work of the Incarnation itself was thus foreshadowed, for as we read (Philippians 2:7), The Son of God "was made in the likeness of men." And again, the glory that is spiritual was anticipated in the angels by way of similitude; and that of the body in the heaven, especially the empyrean. Hence it is written (Ecclesiastes 1:10), "Nothing under the sun is new, for it hath already gone before, in the ages that were before us."[249]

One of the puzzles for us in seeking to understand compatibility between the evolution of the species and the Christian doctrine of creation is the view of original sin and its effects. To the effects of original sin are attributed not just the fallen nature of mankind and our desire to dominate and possess the other, but also the effects on our environment. So, for instance, Thomas Aquinas believed that prior to original sin poisonous animals would have not have injured man. He writes:

> And since then before he sins he would have used the things of this world conformably to the order designed, poisonous animals would not have injured him.

---

[249] Aquinas, *Summa Theologica I*, Q. 73, Art. 1.

In this he does not seem to be saying that the animals were different from the way they are now, rather it seems to be that he is saying that man would have better understood the purposes of such animals and not have used them in such a way that they would have caused harm to him. Following this logic, it is not that there would not have been natural disasters like tsunami, earthquakes or typhoons, but rather that man would have understood them and lived in harmony with them. St Augustine also sought to explain the effects of the Fall by saying that the thorns and thistles were present from the beginning. It is just that man would not have experienced their harm until after the Fall when he had to labour in the fields where they were.[250]

However the *Catechism* has it that:

> The harmony in which they had found themselves, thanks to original justice, is now destroyed: the control of the soul's spiritual faculties over the body is shattered; the union of man and woman becomes subject to tensions, their relations henceforth marked by lust and domination. Harmony with creation is broken: visible creation has become alien and hostile to man. Because of man, creation is now subject "to its bondage to decay". Finally, the consequence explicitly foretold for this disobedience will come true: man will "return to the ground", for out of it he was taken. *Death makes its entrance into human history.*[251]

The authoritative text given for this quote is Genesis 3:16-19:

> To the woman he said, "I will make your pains in childbearing very severe; with painful labor you will give birth to children. Your desire will be for your husband, and he will rule over you." To Adam he said, "Because

---
250 St Augustine, *The Literal Meanings of Genesis*, op. cit., vol. 1, bk. 2, chapter 8.
251 *Catechism of the Catholic Church*, n. 400.

you listened to your wife and ate fruit from the tree about which I commanded you, 'You must not eat from it,' cursed is the ground because of you; through painful toil you will eat food from it all the days of your life. It will produce thorns and thistles for you, and you will eat the plants of the field. By the sweat of your brow you will eat your food until you return to the ground, since from it you were taken; for dust you are and to dust you will return."

The authoritative text for death being the result of their sin is Genesis 2:17: "but you must not eat from the tree of the knowledge of good and evil, for when you eat from it you will certainly die."

These matters are referred to by St Paul when in Romans 8:20-21 he writes:

For the creation was subjected to frustration, not by its own choice, but by the will of the one who subjected it, in hope that the creation itself will be liberated from its bondage to decay and brought into the freedom and glory of the children of God.

8.7 Sin, the Fall and the Sacramentality of All Creation

The sacraments are of central importance to us because they are visible signs of the presence of God. A sacramental vision "sees" God in all things: in all creation and thus in the cosmos, in nature, in history, in material objects, in rocks, plants and trees and especially in ourselves as human persons, who are fashioned in the image and likeness of God. Evolutionary theory particularly links us to the rest of creation by having us emerge within it.

Sin and the Fall affected our relationship to the rest of creation. We became a source of disorder and disharmony, losing our understanding of the Creator and, consequentially, of how we should live in harmony with the divine plan for us and for all creation.

This does not alter the sacramental reality of the created order and the way in which it reflects the divine nature. As Richard McBrien states:

> In this sacramental perspective, all creation is good, even though fallen by sin. Creation is good, first, because it comes from the hand of God and is permeated even now with God's sanctifying presence. At the end of the sixth day of creation, Genesis says, "God saw everything that he had made, and indeed, it was very good" (Gen 1:31).
>
> All creation is good, secondly, because it has been redeemed by the death and resurrection of Christ. "If Christ has not been raised," St. Paul writes, "your faith is futile and you are still in your sins ..." (1 Corinthians 15:17).
>
> Creation is good, thirdly, because it has been renewed and sanctified by the Holy Spirit. "But you are not in the flesh," St. Paul insists, "you are in the Spirit, since the Spirit of God dwells in you" (1 Corinthians 8, 9).
>
> All creation is good, finally, because it has been destined by God for eternal glory. St. Paul writes to the Romans: "For the creation waits with eager longing for the revealing of the children of God ... [for it] will be set free from its bondage to decay and will obtain the freedom of the glory of the children of God" (8:19, 21).[252]

St Paul teaches that the material world and man have a common destiny:

> For the creation waits with eager longing for the revealing of the sons of God ... in hope because the creation itself will be set free from its bondage to decay ... We know that the whole creation has been groaning in travail together

---

[252] Richard McBrien, 'Sacramentality: A Basic Vision for All', *30 Good Minutes*, program 4214, Chicago Sunday Evening Club, 10 January 1999, retrieved from http://www.csec.org/csec/sermon/McBrien_4214.htm (accessed 2010-2014).

until now; and not only the creation, but we ourselves, who have the first fruits of the Spirit, groan inwardly as we wait for adoption as sons, the redemption of our bodies.[253]

The *Catechism*, quoting St Irenaeus, holds that:

> The visible universe, then, is itself destined to be transformed, "so that the world itself, restored to its original state, facing no further obstacles, should be at the service of the just," sharing their glorification in the risen Jesus Christ.[254]

The Second Vatican Council was careful to explain the significance of the Earth for us:

> [Though] we are warned that it profits a man nothing if he gain the whole world and lose himself, the expectation of a new earth must not weaken but rather stimulate our concern for cultivating this one. For here grows the body of a new human family, a body which even now is able to give some kind of foreshadowing of the new age.
>
> Hence, while earthly progress must be carefully distinguished from the growth of Christ's kingdom, to the extent that the former can contribute to the better ordering of human society, it is of vital concern to the Kingdom of God.
>
> For after we have obeyed the Lord, and in His Spirit nurtured on earth the values of human dignity, brotherhood and freedom, and indeed all the good fruits of our nature and enterprise, we will find them again, but freed of stain, burnished and transfigured, when Christ hands over to the Father: "a kingdom eternal and universal, a kingdom of truth and life, of holiness and grace, of justice, love and peace." On this earth that Kingdom is already present in mystery. When the Lord returns it will be brought into full flower.[255]

---

253 Rom 8:19-23
254 *Catechism of the Catholic Church*, n. 1047.
255 Second Vatican Council, *Gaudium et Spes*, op. cit., n. 39.

When we celebrate the seven sacraments, we celebrate the Divine presence. All creation is also a celebration of the Creator, so evident in all that He has made. Creation reflects His goodness and His love. All creation is a sign of God's love.

9
"Brother Wolf": Kinship with Other Species

9.1 Introduction

My little bird sisters, you owe much to God your Creator, and you must always and everywhere praise Him, because He has given you the freedom to fly anywhere – also He has given you a double and triple covering, and your colourful and pretty clothing, and your food is ready without your working for it, and your singing that was taught to you by the Creator, and your numbers that have been multiplied by the blessing of God – and because He preserved your species in Noah's ark so that your race should not disappear from the earth. And you are also indebted to Him for the realm of the air which He assigned to you. Moreover, you neither sow nor reap, yet God nourishes you, and He gives you the rivers and springs to drink from. He gives you high mountains and hills, rocks and crags as refuges, and lofty trees in which to make your nests. And although you do not know how to spin or sow, God gives you and your little ones the clothing which you need. So the Creator loves you very much, since He gives you so many good things. Therefore my little bird sisters, be careful not to be ungrateful, but strive always to praise God.[256]

St Francis of Assisi and many other saints, especially those

---

256 Francis of Assisi, *Little Flowers of St Francis*, trans. R. Brown, New York, Doubleday, 1991, pp. 76-77.

who were wanderers or hermits, had a special relationship to wild animals – a piety which took many forms including appreciation, love and rescue- and an understanding of animals as fellow creatures and of the environment as reflecting God's love and providence for them. The hagiographies record that the relationships were often reciprocal with animals showing special regard for the saints and appearing to grieve when they died. The saints often referred to animals as their followers or disciples and not just their companions.

That was all prior to contemporary knowledge of molecular biology and contemporary theories of evolution which indicate a great closeness of humans to the animal kingdom. The idea that we emerged from animals and from even earlier forms of life connects us to the animal kingdom in a way that the saints may have expressed but could not have known. Our biological connectedness to the animal kingdom prompts us to think about what separates us from animals.

Some contemporary writers, such as Peter Singer,[257] suggest that we should consider animal suffering on the same level as human suffering. Singer goes further claiming that because some animals have a higher level of functioning than some humans they may even be of greater moral status than some humans. A newborn infant, while much loved by his or her parents, may not have the capacity yet for understanding which may be expressed by a dolphin or an African grey parrot or an elephant. As Christians we answer claims of this nature on the grounds that the newborn infant is of a kind of being that has the inherent capacity for intelligence beyond that which can be expressed by the dolphin, the parrot or the elephant. Further, as a matter of faith we recognize that the newborn infant is made in the image and likeness of God.

---

[257] Peter Singer, *Practical Ethics*, 2nd, Cambridge, Cambridge University Press, 1993.

Significantly, the infant belongs to the human family, which indicates his or her interrelatedness, and the infant is rightly the recipient of human love.

That still leaves, however, the matter of animal suffering even if we do not give animals the same status as humans. To what extent does the suffering of an animal matter? To what extent should we be concerned about the slaughter of animals, especially the gratuitous slaughter of animals for sport rather than for food or clothing? There are also questions about the preservation of whole species and whether we should be concerned about a species going into extinction, and related questions about the destruction of environments and habitats for animals.

These are questions that do need to be addressed even if we do not share the same piety that some of the saints expressed in their relationships to animals.

9.2 Peter Singer's Criticisms

Singer is highly critical of Christianity in relation to the treatment of animals within the Christian tradition.[258] He claims that Jesus never really addressed the question of our relationship to animals and refers critically to the passage in Mark's gospel in which Jesus casts out demons by sending them into pigs which then promptly are drowned:

> They went across the lake to the region of the Gerasenes. When Jesus got out of the boat, a man with an impure spirit came from the tombs to meet him. This man lived in the tombs, and no one could bind him anymore, not even with a chain. For he had often been chained hand and foot, but he tore the chains apart and broke the irons on his feet. No one was strong enough to subdue him. Night and

---

258 Singer, *In Defense of Animals*, op. cit.

day among the tombs and in the hills he would cry out and cut himself with stones. When he saw Jesus from a distance, he ran and fell on his knees in front of him. He shouted at the top of his voice, "What do you want with me, Jesus, Son of the Most High God? In God's name don't torture me!" For Jesus had said to him, "Come out of this man, you impure spirit!" Then Jesus asked him, "What is your name?" "My name is Legion," he replied, "for we are many." And he begged Jesus again and again not to send them out of the area. A large herd of pigs was feeding on the nearby hillside. The demons begged Jesus, "Send us among the pigs; allow us to go into them." He gave them permission, and the impure spirits came out and went into the pigs. The herd, about two thousand in number, rushed down the steep bank into the lake and were drowned (Mark 5:1-13).

Referring to Genesis and the *imago Dei*, Singer claims that Christianity gives a protected status to human beings alone. He quotes St Augustine:

> Christ himself shows that to refrain from the killing of animals and the destroying of plants is the height of superstition, for judging that there are no common rights between us and the beast and trees, he sent the devils into a herd of swine ... Surely the swine had not sinned, nor had the tree.[259]

Singer claims that the Christian view of the special and uniquely protected status of human beings has been challenged in recent times. First, there have been the effects of the development of an understanding of evolution and the evidence for it which he claims is incompatible with the creation view. Second, he refers to the

---

259 St Augustine, *The Catholic and Manichaean Ways of Life, The Fathers of the Church: A New Translation* vol. 56, trans. D.A. Gallagher and I.J. Gallagher, Boston, Catholic University Press, 1966, p. 102. (cf. Singer, *Practical Ethics*, p. 240).

arguments of those who claim that selecting humans as always superior to non-human animals is in error, especially in relation to the great apes whose activities indicate considerable intelligence. He argues that the biology suggests that we are very close to the great apes, belonging to the same family, and so have little reason to claim a uniquely protected status and that our treatment of animals is a kind of racism, what he has called "speciesism". Third, he claims that in recent times there has been growth in the knowledge that there are animals that show greater intelligence than some humans.[260]

Singer also has a discussion of what is meant by "person" and applies the Christian use of the word to a non-human as it relates to the persons of the Blessed Trinity. On that basis he argues that the word person is not exclusive to human beings. He refers to the philosopher Boethius who redefined a person as "an individual substance of a rational nature". He uses this definition to argue that because some animals, such as the great apes, display intelligence and some humans do not, such as those who are severely disabled developmentally including infants with anencephaly, the concept of person may not include all humans and could include some animals.[261]

Singer argues that our ideas of equality in relation to racism and sexism are not based on arguing that there are no differences between races or differences of gender. If someone were to show for instance that men and women have quite different attributes and even different abilities this would not justify sexism; those who partake in the race wars in trying to argue that some races are intellectually inferior have missed the point. The point is that all human beings are of equal status and equally worthy of respect, whatever their level of ability. He writes:

---
260 Singer, *In Defense of Animals*, op. cit.
261 Ibid.

The appropriate response to those who claim to have found evidence of genetically based differences in ability between the races or sexes is not to stick to the belief that the genetic explanation must be wrong, what other evidence to the contrary may turn up: instead we should make it quite clear that the claim to equality does not depend on intelligence, moral capacity, physical strength, or similar matters of fact. Equality is a moral ideal, not a simple assertion of fact. There is no logically compelling reason for assuming that a factual difference in ability between two people justifies any difference in the amount of consideration we give to satisfying the needs and interests. The principle of the equality of human beings is not a description of an alleged actual equality among humans: it is a prescription of how we should treat humans.[262]

Peter Singer's basic approach to morality is utilitarian. He identifies himself as a preference utilitarian. Utilitarianism has its basis in the universalization of desires or preferences. Preferences or desires are prescriptive in that they contain or imply a prescription for their fulfilment. Universalizability is a logical principle that holds that one is committed to making the same moral judgment in relevantly similar circumstances. In other words it is a principle of consistency. If you apply it to the preferences that people choose then utilitarians hold that the principle results in the idea that we should maximize the satisfaction of preferences. This idea is simply a matter of equality. Each person counts for one and no-one for more than one. The nature of preferences is that we seek to satisfy them and this provides the prescriptive content for a moral system that then applies a principle of universality to preferences.

The satisfaction of preferences then applies equally to the

---

[262] Peter Singer, 'All Animals Are Equal', in *Applied Ethics*, New York, Oxford University Press, 1988, pp. 219-220.

animal kingdom as it does to the human realm with some animals having preferences and some humans not. Pleasure and pain are of equal consideration no matter who or what is the subject.

On the basis of a principle of equality, which he refers to as a principle of equal consideration of interests, Singer argues that we have no basis for not taking into account the interests of any creature that is capable of suffering pain. He writes:

> If a being suffers, there can be no moral justification for refusing to take that suffering into consideration. No matter what the nature of the being, the principle of equality requires that its suffering be counted equally with the like suffering – insofar as rough comparisons can be made – of any other being. If it is a being that is not capable of suffering, or experiencing enjoyment or happiness, there is nothing to be taken into account.[263]

He argues, on that basis, that sentience, the capacity for consciousness and for feeling pain, is the only defensible boundary of concern to the interests of others and to mark that boundary by some characteristic like intelligence or rationality would be arbitrary.[264]

On that basis he argues that our practices in relation to slaughtering and killing animals for food, and research on animals, especially practices such as vivisection, are unjustifiable because we have no reason for regarding animal suffering as any less significant than human suffering. On the grounds that any satisfactory defence of the claim that all and only humans have intrinsic dignity, he challenges those who postulate human dignity as differentiating humans from animals to refer, as a necessity, to some relevant capacities or characteristics that all and only

---
263 Ibid., p. 222.
264 Ibid.

humans possess. This then leads to the problem that some animals possess human characteristics, such as intelligence, more than some humans.[265]

9.3 *Imago Dei*

The basis of Peter Singer's dismissal of a Christian view of our being made in the image and likeness of God and of our unique place within creation is his concept of the equal consideration of interests which he bases on desires or preferences and the capacity to feel pain or to experience happiness. He makes no pretence to a metaphysical view of human nature.

The Christian view of human nature includes the notion that we are made for a purpose, made to love God and to be loved by God. We understand human beings as being inherently social and Christian morality as being based on the concept of love as complete gift of self. St Thomas Aquinas explained that the ultimate goal of human existence is union and eternal communion with God. This is referred to as the *beatific vision*, in which a person is to experience perfect unending happiness by seeing the very essence of God. He taught that the beatific vision occurs after death, as a gift from God given to those who have experienced salvation and redemption through Christ while living on earth. Through Christ, who has redeemed us from sin, we also seek to participate in that Divine life in this life. We do so by ordering our will toward the right things, such as love, peace, and holiness. Those who truly seek to understand and see God will necessarily love what God loves.[266]

Peter Singer has a point in relation to the way in which we regard animal suffering. We have little reason to treat animal suf-

---

[265] Ibid., p. 228.
[266] Aquinas, *Summa Theologica I:II*, Q. 3, Art 6.

fering differently from human suffering if animal suffering is no different from human suffering. A question to ask would be whether the suffering of animals can be compared to human suffering because so much of our experience of suffering is anticipatory. Part of our experience of suffering is fear of future suffering and the experience of pain is, in part, fear of disability or the actual experience of disability as well as the pain itself. In other words a being that is self-conscious and intelligent would seem to have a greater capacity to suffer than a being that experienced pain but had little capacity to see itself existing into the future or to have the abstract thoughts which are part of the pain experience for a human. We can therefore differentiate between pain and suffering in self-conscious beings who can think abstractly, wonder and fear for the future and beings whose suffering is restricted to the moment.

Suffering, pleasure and pain are not the only issues. An issue that Peter Singer does not address in his chapter on animals is the issue of killing. He discusses suffering, and suffering associated with slaughter, but not the issue of the taking of a life.

We might be willing to concede that, as a matter of equality, the suffering of an animal should be taken into account to the extent that it is a similar experience to human suffering. We would therefore be concerned about farming and slaughter practices to ensure that they do not cause suffering in animals, but it is a different matter to claim that the taking of an animal life is of the same order as the taking of a human life.

Singer would want to argue that if we consider human life to be inviolable or sacred, we need to appeal to some feature or characteristic that makes human life different, and if we do that we are likely to encounter the same problem which is that there will be some animals that possess those characteristics to a greater extent than some humans.

The issue in this for Christians is relational, in the sense that our morality is based on the idea of our relationship to God and our relationship to neighbour. The *imago Dei* sets human beings apart, as does the Incarnation, because it indicates a special place for human beings in God's plan of creation. To kill a human being is to kill a person made in the image and likeness of God. It is an act that *in itself* cannot be oriented towards God because it is the destruction of someone God loves and who has been created to love God.

Philosophically, we give an account of human beings as Boethius did in terms of an animal that has a rational nature. Though there is indication of relatively intelligent behaviour on the part of some animals, such as the great apes or dolphins or the African grey parrot, there does seem to be a gulf between the capacity of a normal adult human being and the capacity of the most intelligent of animals. One of the features that separates us from animals is language. Animals can communicate, with sounds that have an intelligible meaning, to each other. Parrots can mimic the sounds of language but that is a far cry from the expression of abstract thoughts. An animal would seem to completely lack the capacity to have an understanding of the divine. Human beings would seem to be uniquely placed in being able to return God's love. Animals can express affection for each other and, as pets, for their masters but there is no evidence that they could conceive of a god or wonder about the mystery of creation.

Therefore we would seem to be justified in treating a human life as radically different from an animal life because of our inherent intellectual capacity. As Christians our morality is relational in that it is based on love of God and love of neighbour. The issue of human beings who lack intellectual capacity, either through immaturity, lack of development or through illness or disease, is easily understood in the context in which we recognize human beings as having an inherent capacity for intellectual life even if, for some reason, that capacity remains dormant or has been suppressed. Being the fruit of human generation and having a human genome provides us with the capacity to develop an intellectual life. However it also makes us a member of the human family, that is, the family of individuals who have the capacity for an intellectual life. When we see a human being, we see a member of our family who is properly the subject of our love.

As a theological matter, we understand that in being made in the image and likeness of God we have been given an immortal soul. This also places us in a different category from the non-human animals. We have stewardship of all creation and within that we have a particular stewardship over human life because we are made in the image and likeness of God and have an immortal soul. St Augustine deals with this question as part of a discussion of suicide and the commandment not to kill. He writes:

> And so some attempt to extend this command even to beasts and cattle, as if it forbade us to take life from any creature. But if so, why not extend it also to the plants, and all that is rooted in and nourished by the earth? For though this class of creatures have no sensation, yet they also are said to live, and consequently they can die; and therefore, if violence be done them, can be killed. So, too, the apostle, when speaking of the seeds of such things as these, says, That which you sow is not quickened except it die; and in the Psalm it is said, He killed their vines with hail. Must we therefore reckon it a breaking of this commandment, You shall not kill, to pull a flower? Are we thus insanely to countenance the foolish error of the Manichæans? Putting aside, then, these ravings, if, when we say, You shall not kill, we do not understand this of the plants, since they have no sensation, nor of the irrational animals that fly, swim, walk, or creep, since

they are dissociated from us by their want of reason, and are therefore by the just appointment of the Creator subjected to us to kill or keep alive for our own uses; if so, then it remains that we understand that commandment simply of man. The commandment is, You shall not kill man; therefore neither another nor yourself, for he who kills himself still kills nothing else than man.[267]

9.4 Evolution, Microbiology and Kinship

Understanding human beings as the pinnacle of an evolutionary process does have an impact on the way in which we regard animals; that they are constructed in very much the same way as we are, having very similar genetic structures to our own and sharing ancestry does link them to us in a way that the saints and the ancients might not have conceived. When we see an animal exhibiting signs of pain or frustration we can not only see a likeness to our own experience of pain or frustration, we also know that physiologically their mechanisms for experiencing pain are very similar to our own. This awareness ought to make us concerned about animal suffering. Jame Schaefer writes of our origins:

> Although the evidence for the evolution and nature of our species was gathered by palaeontologists, comparative anatomists, embryologists, and biogeographers during the latter half of the 19th and early 20th centuries, several other disciplines – including genetics, cell biology, physiology, and ecology – yielded new knowledge during the first half of the 20th century that can only be understood within the framework of the scientific theory of evolution. The birth and blossoming of molecular biology during the second half of the 20th century provided convincing evidence of biological evolution and the means to recon-

---

[267] St Augustine, *City of God*, bk. 1, chapter 20.

struct evolutionary history of living organisms with detail and precision.[268]

Though comparisons can be made between humans and the non-human primates, in that the latter are socially organized, can be taught limited forms of symbolic communication and have some self-awareness, as discussed earlier, normal adult humans have a self-consciousness which seems to be without parallel amongst the other primates, humans have a greater capacity to remember the past, to anticipate the future, to use abstract symbols and to imagine possibilities and events that are unrelated to our present experience. Human beings are usually aware of their mortality and are able to reflect on their origins and whether their lives have purpose. Perhaps the most significant aspect of being human that separates us from animals is our capacity to have a moral life and to shape the kind of character that we choose to be by the decisions that we make. In other words we alone of the created order have true freedom. Perhaps most significantly for a believer is our capacity for divine grace, particularly the grace of deification that unites us to God, to which we are open in this life and hope to receive in the next life. We are made in the image of God but our tradition holds that we have the capacity, with divine assistance, to become like God in a passive process ultimately of kenosis[269] in which we become united with the Creator, having surrendered in dying all that we are bound to in this life.[270]

---

268 Schaefer, op. cit., p. 167.

269 In Christian tradition, "kenosis" is the 'self-emptying' of one's own will and becoming entirely conformed to God's divine will. The Scriptural source for it is in St Paul's letter to the Philippians 2:7

270 I am a philosopher not a theologian, but fascinated by theological analysis. I am deeply indebted to the account of deification produced by my colleague Adam Cooper in his *Naturally Human, Supernaturally God: Deification in Pre-conciliar Catholicism* (Fortress Press: US 2014), in which he compares three pre-conciliar accounts of deification. From his analysis I came to more deeply appreciate the significance of deification as a passive reception of divine grace to which we only have to be open, not something that we actually achieve. We can create barriers to divine like-

Some have argued for what is called sociobiology, the idea that moral behaviour itself has evolved in the sense that human communities and individuals who developed standards of moral behaviour were more likely to survive to reproduce than communities that were unable to establish any kind of moral social contract.[271] A mistake that can be made, on the basis that moral capacity evolved, is to argue that the kinds of social behaviours that would favour survival are therefore morally preferred.

The term seems to have been coined by Edward Wilson.[272] Sociobiology is criticised for genetic determinism, which attributes human behaviours to inherited characteristics rather than the combination of culture and reason. It may be the case that our capacity to reason and to decide to adopt values that are needed for living in community evolved. One could well imagine that natural selection would favour communities of people who were able to

---

ness through sin, or even by preventing kenotic surrender through attachments, even love, which fails to recognize the priority of surrendering to the divine, everything and everyone that are important to us. I have found that kenosis a source of great grief and tragedy in my own life, as I contemplate losing the relationships of those I love in that final lonely journey to my own death and the difficulty of being willing to surrender all that I love here on earth. But Adam's account explains that that is not something I do but instead receive passively through being open to the work of God, through his grace within me uniting me to him in my willingness to surrender. The end of life can be a battle to survive against the rigours of disease processes. Deification allows us to see that as the work of God within us to which we only need to be passively receptive. Deification and kenosis are not our achievement but God's. Our contribution is not to hinder deification by refusing to surrender those relationships that in this life are so important to us. In that there is trust, joy and great sadness. This in fact is the theme of C.S. Lewis's whimsical writing, entitled, *The Great Divorce*. Heaven awaits those who have no barriers to the way of divine grace: barriers including not just unrepented sin but also attachment to that which we love in this life. In the end we are carried across the abyss alone by God's grace and not by anything of our own doing. Those close to us are unlikely to want us to surrender, but to continue the battle to live in their love. But, in death, we must surrender to God's will for which we were created.

271 Janet Radcliffe Richards, *Human Nature After Darwin: A Philosophical Introduction*, London, Routledge, 2000.
272 E.O. Wilson, *Sociobiology: The New Synthesis*, Cambridge, Mass., Harvard University Press, 1975.

live in relational community, but that tells us nothing about the worth or value of particular moral choices.

To his credit, Richard Dawkins in his book *The Selfish Gene* rejects using evolutionary theory as a basis for morality:

> A human society based simply on the genes law of universal ruthless selfishness would be a very nasty society in which to live. But unfortunately, however much we may deplore something, it does not stop it being true. This book is mainly intended to be interesting, but if you would extract a moral from it, read it as a warning. Be warned that if you wish, as I do, to build a society in which individuals cooperate generously and unselfishly towards a common good, you can expect little help from biological nature. Let us try to teach generosity and altruism, because we are born selfish. That is we understand what our own selfish genes are up to, because we may then at least have the chance to upset their designs, something that no other species has ever aspired to.[273]

If it is the case that the capacity for moral behaviour evolved, that is the evolution of the capacity to reason and to recognize the rightful claims of others, this does not specify what the content of morality should be. The latter is a matter of applying our capacity for reason. There is a danger that sociobiology leads to a kind of moral determinism and that should be avoided.

The kind of morality that evolution produces is a very unattractive one; it is based on competing for physical survival and security in which love is no more than a social contract for mutual survival advantages, rather than a real emotion which has the interests of another genuinely at heart.

However our evolutionary, molecular and genetic kinship does give us reason to pause and reflect on our common creatureliness.

---

273 Dawkins, *The Selfish Gene*, op. cit., p. 3.

With the animals we are made by God and we share the resources of the universe that God has given us with them. If we are to reflect on peace and harmony within creation as God's will for us, then the way in which we treat the animal kingdom is of significance.

9.5 The Saints

This brings us back to the saints, such as St. Francis, who developed unusual attitudes towards animals including forming relationships with them. According to Roger Sorrell, Francis's attitude to animals was a part of the chivalry that had developed at the time. He understood that God's relationship to creation was one of gratuitous benefits to both the just and the unjust. He saw that our godliness should also express itself in chivalry to all of God's creation. So in a sense he had spiritualized the chivalric values of the time of largesse and noblesse oblige, particularly deference to others especially those in lower stations. His ideas of chivalry occurred at three levels: between God and humanity, between humans, and between humankind and the rest of creation. Chivalry, on the part of God, is condescending love to those both unjust and just, the chosen and the unchosen. God's chivalry is a sister to God's love. In dealing with his fellow human beings Francis had the chivalric notion that almsgiving reflected well on both the donor and the recipient. The notion of chivalry extended to the proper use of divine creation and the acceptance of God's beneficence to human beings in creating animals.[274]

The notion of chivalry that St. Francis expressed was consistent with using animals for food. He rejected the extreme asceticism of the Cathars who were vegetarians though they were prepared to eat fish, believing that fish were not propagated by coitus. His

---

[274] R.D. Sorrell, *St Francis of Assisi and Nature: Tradition and Innovation in Western Christian Attitudes Towards the Environment*, Oxford, Oxford University Press, 1988, pp. 69-74.

acceptance of eating animals seems to have been based on St. Paul's letter to Timothy which affirms that everything created by God is good and nothing is to be rejected if it is received with thanksgiving because it is sanctified by the Word of God and prayer.[275]

> The Spirit clearly says that in later times some will abandon the faith and follow deceiving spirits and things taught by demons. Such teachings come through hypocritical liars, whose consciences have been seared as with a hot iron. They forbid people to marry and order them to abstain from certain foods, which God created to be received with thanksgiving by those who believe and who know the truth. For everything God created is good, and nothing is to be rejected if it is received with thanksgiving, because it is consecrated by the word of God and prayer (1 Timothy 4:1-5).

A further element of St Francis's relationship to all creation is often described as his nature mysticism. Nature mysticism has been defined in terms of being based on an idea of Christian beliefs that involve an appreciation that creation is God's handiwork. Sorrell describes a nature mystical experience as one which arises when a positive conception of the beauty and worth of creation, and its intimate relationship with a spiritual force of some sort, catalyses profound personal reactions of wonder or exhilaration. In the face of an overwhelming encounter with the sublimity of the natural world in general, the mystic progresses directly towards a vision of, contact with, or participation in that spiritual force.[276]

The mysticism of St. Francis is described poignantly in an episode in which he is reported chatting to the creatures with inward and outward joy, just as if they felt, understood, and could

---

275 Ibid., p. 75.
276 Ibid., p. 82.

talk about God. Many times, in this way, he became wrapped in contemplation of God.[277] The *Sermon on the Birds* and the *Canticle of the Sun* and many other reports of his nature mysticism seem to indicate a real relationship with nature in which he spoke to creatures as though they could understand and warranted the same chivalry with which he treated his fellow human beings. One such story is reported to have taken place when he was presented with a fish on the Lake of Rieti.

> He accepted it joyfully and kindly and began to call it brother; and placing it in the water outside the boat, he began devoutly to bless the name of the Lord. And he continued in prayer for some time, while the fish played in the water beside the boat, and did not go away from the place where it had been put until his prayer was finished ...[278]

Sorrell writes that the sources positively light up with emotional phrases when they come to the subject of Francis's feelings. They referred to Francis having feelings of unheard-of devotion to creatures – his joy, love, rapture, and adoration of the divine in creation. In these accounts there is an emphasis on the honest, simple, human sexual and emotional beginning of the mystical experience in the path taken by Francis.[279]

The Canticle of the Sun deserves a special place of mention for its importance and significance for the church:

> Most High, all-powerful, all-good Lord,
> All praise is Yours, all glory, honor and blessings.
> To you alone, Most High, do they belong;
> no mortal lips are worthy to pronounce Your Name.

---

277 Ibid., p. 94.
278 Ibid., p. 95.
279 Ibid., p. 96.

"Brother Wolf": Kinship with Other Species

We praise You, Lord, for all Your creatures,
especially for Brother Sun,
who is the day through whom You give us light.
And he is beautiful and radiant with great splendor,
of You Most High, he bears your likeness.
We praise You, Lord, for Sister Moon and the stars,
in the heavens you have made them bright, precious and fair.
We praise You, Lord, for Brothers Wind and Air,
 fair and stormy, all weather's moods,
by which You cherish all that You have made.
We praise You, Lord, for Sister Water,
so useful, humble, precious and pure.
We praise You, Lord, for Brother Fire,
through whom You light the night.
He is beautiful, playful, robust, and strong.
We praise You, Lord, for Sister Earth,
who sustains us
with her fruits, colored flowers, and herbs.
We praise You, Lord, for those who pardon,
for love of You bear sickness and trial.
Blessed are those who endure in peace,
by You Most High, they will be crowned.
We praise You, Lord, for Sister Death,
from whom no-one living can escape.
Woe to those who die in their sins!
Blessed are those that She finds doing Your Will.
No second death can do them harm.
We praise and bless You, Lord, and give You thanks,
and serve You in all humility.

There have been many controversies about the interpretation of the Canticle. First there were arguments over whether Francis is giving praise to God for the sun and the moon or whether instead he is calling on the sun and the moon to praise God. The latter is a much more mystical interpretation. He is reported to have made his own commentary about his intention to write the Canticle:

> Therefore, for his glory, for my consolation, and the edification of my neighbour I wish to compose a new praise of the Lord concerning His creatures. These creatures minister to our needs every day; without them we could not live; and through them the human race greatly offends the creator. Every day we fail to appreciate so great a blessing by not raising as we should the creator and dispenser of all these gifts.[280]

The commentator, Sorrell, reporting this explanation says that Francis sat down and concentrated and then cried out: "Most high, all-powerful, and good Lord."[281]

The Canticle was written over a number of years with the last and second last stanzas being added later. The first part in praise of the beauty and holiness of nature as a reflection of the Divine was written in the Spring of 1225, immediately after he received the stigmata during an extended meditation retreat among some caves.[282]

The second section, the segment on forgiveness and peace, was composed soon after hearing and in response to the squabbling of political and religious authorities in Assisi. The final verses were written late the following year as St. Francis was dying, a time in which he seems to be welcoming "sister death".[283]

---

280 Ibid., p. 119.
281 Ibid.
282 Ivan M. Granger, 'The Canticle of Brother Sun', *Poetry Chaikhana*, retrieved from http://www.poetry-chaikhana.com/F/FrancisofAsi/CanticleofBr.htm (accessed 6 August 2011).
283 Ibid.

St Thomas Aquinas had a more utilitarian approach to animals. He is often quoted as saying that cruelty to animals is only evil because it disposes to cruelty to humans. However the passage is more nuanced than this would suggest:

> Affection in man is twofold: it may be an affection of reason, or it may be an affection of passion. If a man's affection be one of reason, it matters not how man behaves to animals, because God has subjected all things to man's power, according to Psalm 8:8: "Thou hast subjected all things under his feet": and it is in this sense that the Apostle says that "God has no care for oxen"; because God does not ask of man what he does with oxen or other animals.
>
> But if man's affection be one of passion, then it is moved also in regard to other animals: for since the passion of pity is caused by the afflictions of others; and since it happens that even irrational animals are sensible to pain, it is possible for the affection of pity to arise in a man with regard to the sufferings of animals. Now it is evident that if a man practice a pitiful affection for animals, he is all the more disposed to take pity on his fellow-men: wherefore it is written (Proverbs 11:10): "The just regardeth the lives of his beasts: but the bowels of the wicked are cruel." Consequently the Lord, in order to inculcate pity to the Jewish people, who were prone to cruelty, wished them to practice pity even with regard to dumb animals, and forbade them to do certain things savoring of cruelty to animals. Hence He prohibited them to "boil a kid in the milk of its dam"; and to "muzzle the ox that treadeth out the corn"; and to slay "the dam with her young." It may, nevertheless, be also said that these prohibitions were made in hatred of idolatry. For the Egyptians held it to be wicked to allow the ox to eat of the grain while threshing the corn.

Moreover certain sorcerers were wont to ensnare the mother bird with her young during incubation, and to employ them for the purpose of securing fruitfulness and good luck in bringing up children: also because it was held to be a good omen to find the mother sitting on her young.[284]

Nevertheless his approach is a far cry from that of St Francis.

9.6 Conclusion

Francis had a special relationship to creation: he not only recognized and celebrated God's gifts to us in all creation, but he also communicated with God's creation, humbling himself by calling them brother or sister. He may be relatively unique in preaching to the animals and have them reportedly respond to his ministry, but he is not alone in our tradition in finding evidence of the Creator in creation. Psalm 19 contains the words:

> The heavens are telling the glory of God; and the firmament proclaims his handiwork. Day to day pours forth speech, and night to night declares knowledge. There is no speech, nor are there words; their voice is not heard; yet their voice goes out through all the earth, and their words to the end of the world. In them he has set a tent for the sun, which comes forth like a bridegroom leaving his chamber, and like a strong man runs its course with joy. Its rising is from the end of the heavens, and its circuit to the end of them; and there is nothing hid from its heat (Ps 19:1-6).

We are part of divine creation, an extraordinary part, in which we, uniquely of the species, have knowledge of God and the capacity to love. However, all creation is affected by our sin and all creation is redeemed by the life, suffering, death and resurrection of Jesus. We are given a role of stewardship for which we are to be

---
284 Aquinas, *Summa Theologica I:II*, Q. 102, Art. 6, Obj. 8.

held to account. The other animals are our responsibility and their suffering is a matter that we should address.

St Thomas Aquinas saw the variety of the various species as reflective of God's goodness:

> For he has brought things forth into being, so as to share his goodness with his creatures, and to represent it through creatures. And because it cannot be adequately represented through one creature, he brought forth many and varied creatures, so that what one creature fails to represent of the divine goodness is supplemented by another. For goodness, which in God is simple and has only one form, is variously present in creatures.[285]

Pope John Paul II wrote about:

> ... [the] appropriateness of acquiring a growing awareness of the fact that one cannot use with impunity the different categories of beings, whether living or inanimate – animals, plants, the natural elements – simply as one wishes, according to one's own economic needs. On the contrary, one must take into account the nature of each being and of its mutual connection in an ordered system, which is precisely the cosmos.[286]

A Christian approach to animals is complex. We appreciate them because they are part of creation and thus a sign of the divine nature and their presence a sign of divine love. We recognize that each creature exists as part of the divine plan, not accidentally or as a result of mere chance.

In respecting and loving the Creator we respect His design and purpose for each creature and seek stewardship of them based on trying to understand what the divine purpose for each creature is and acting in accordance with that purpose.

---

285 Aquinas, *Summa Theologica I*, Q. 47, Art. 1.
286 Pope John Paul II, *Sollicitudo Rei Socialis*, 30 December 1987, n. 34.

IN MEMORIAM

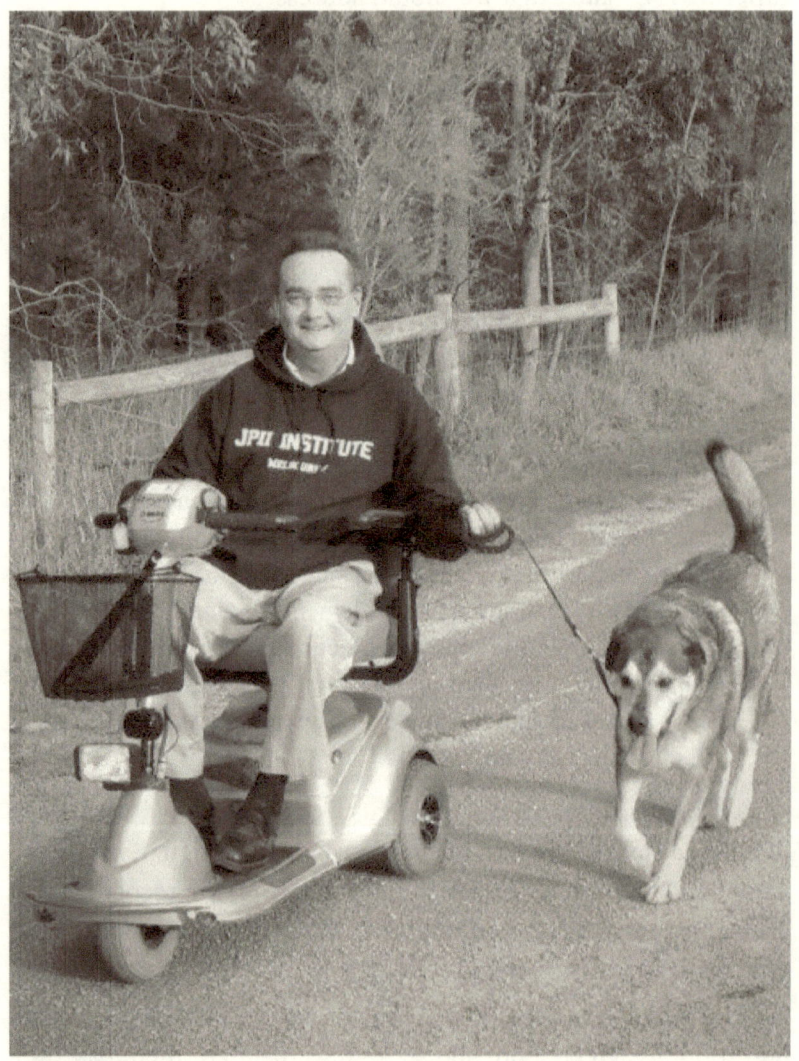

"We are part of divine creation, an extraordinary part, in which we, uniquely of the species, have knowledge of God and the capacity to love. However, all creation is affected by our sin and all creation is redeemed by the life, suffering, death and resurrection of Jesus."

I am a philosopher not a theologian, but fascinated by theological analysis. I am deeply indebted to the account of deification produced by my colleague Adam Cooper in his *Naturally Human, Supernaturally God: Deification in Pre-conciliar Catholicism* (Fortress Press: US 2014), in which he compares three pre-conciliar accounts of deification. From his analysis I came to more deeply appreciate the significance of deification as a passive reception of divine grace to which we only have to be open, not something that we actually achieve. We can create barriers to divine likeness through sin, or even by preventing kenotic surrender through attachments, even love, which fails to recognize the priority of surrendering to the divine, everything and everyone that are important to us. I have found that kenosis a source of great grief and tragedy in my own life, as I contemplate losing the relationships of those I love in that final lonely journey to my own death and the difficulty of being willing to surrender all that I love here on earth. But Adam's account explains that that is not something I do but instead receive passively through being open to the work of God, through his grace within me uniting me to him in my willingness to surrender. The end of life can be a battle to survive against the rigours of disease processes. Deification allows us to see that as the work of God within us to which we only need to be passively receptive. Deification and kenosis are not our achievement but God's. Our contribution is not to hinder deification by refusing to surrender those relationships that in this life are so important to us. In that there is trust, joy and great sadness. This in fact is the theme of C.S. Lewis's whimsical writing, entitled, *The Great Divorce*. Heaven awaits those who have no barriers to the way of divine grace: barriers including not just unrepented sin but also attachment to that which we love in this life. In the end we are carried across the abyss alone by God's grace and not by anything of our own doing. Those close to us are unlikely to want us to surrender, but to continue the battle to live in their love. But, in death, we must surrender to God's will for which we were created.

Nicholas Tonti-Filippini (1956-2014)

AFTERWORD

Bringing this fifth volume of *About Bioethics* "to life", without the author's physical presence, has been a poignant, privileged experience – enriching and challenging – as expected with any project of loving creation.

My heartfelt gratitude goes to Bernadette de Bruyn for agreeing to assist with editing after a long break. I am very much indebted also to our children for their love and support in so many ways – to Justin who contributed significant technical assistance before leaving to study overseas, to Claire who capably stepped in after this, and to Lucianne and John for their constant encouragement and helpful comments throughout the process.

There are many friends and colleagues as well to whom I am grateful – always responding to requests for advice or assistance with generosity and a warmth that has been uplifting.

Of course, my deepest gratitude goes to Nicholas for the inspiration of his ever unfailing love, courage and determination to share with us the wisdom and insights of the marvellous intellect gifted to him by his Creator.

Mary Tonti-Filippini
March 2017

Deo Gratias

Editor's note: These appendices were intended to be chapters. They were written in 2011 and revisited, in part, in 2014 for a lecture series entitled 'Ethics, Creation and the Environment'.

APPENDIX A: THE POPULATION QUESTION

1. Introduction

The date on which this lecture was to be delivered for the first time, 31 October 2011, is the day that the UN forecast that seven billion people would inhabit the earth. 2011's State of World Population report, *People and Possibilities in a World of 7 Billion*, looks at the dynamics behind the numbers. It explains the trends that are defining our world of seven billion and documents actions that people in vastly different countries and circumstances are taking in their own communities to make the most of their, and our, world.[287]

Some of these trends are remarkable: today, 893 million people are 60 or older. By the middle of this century that number will nearly triple, to reach 2.4 billion. About one in two people now live in an urban area. In about 35 years, two out of three will. People are living longer. Today's average life span is 68 years, compared to 48 in 1950.[288]

This indicates that the effective policies to limit fertility and improve health and longevity are creating another problem altogether, especially in countries such as China and the developed countries which have less than replacement birth rates and thus a future demographic in which there may be insufficient workforce to provide the taxes to pay for, and the human resources to provide

---

[287] United Nations Family Planning Association (UNFPA), State of World Population report: *People and Possibilities in a World of 7 Billion*, 2011, retrieved from http://www.unfpa.org/publications/state-world-population-2011 (accessed 2010-2014).
[288] Ibid.

for, care of people with disabilities and older people who are more consumers of services than providers. An economic issue is the proportion of people who are in the workforce compared to those such as children and those who are too ill, disabled or frail to work productively. Although of course technology affects the relative need for labour to achieve improved productivity.

Often poverty is associated with high population growth but, in fact, according to the UN, in 2014, many developing countries have reduced poverty while maintaining high population growth rates.

> If rapid population growth always caused higher poverty, then the last 50 years should have been one of the most impoverishing periods in human history. In fact, it was a period of rising living standards in most of the developing world. Food production per capita increased in most regions, with Africa an important exception. In India, where many feared mass starvation in the 1960s, food production has more than tripled, with a 40% increase in food per capita since 1960. The proportion of the population in poverty declined in most regions. Even Africa, which had rising poverty rates in the 1980s, has had declining poverty rates since the early 1990s. Many countries in Asia and Latin America experienced the fastest improvements in their living standards in history at the same time their populations were growing at historically unprecedented rates.[289]

The UNFPA State of the World Population 2011 report makes the case for planning and investing in people. By empowering people to improve their own lives, we can foster sustainable cities that serve as catalysts for progress, productive labour forces that fuel economic growth, youth populations that contribute to the

---

289 David Lam, 'Population dynamics and poverty in retrospect', *The World We Want*, 2013, http://www.worldwewant2015.org/node/301885 (accessed 28 July 2014).

Appendix A: The Population Question

well-being of economies and societies, and a generation of healthy older people who are actively engaged in the social and economic affairs of their communities.[290]

The effect on the environment of population growth is a factor in sustainability, but other relevant factors for sustainability are per capita consumption and the use of non-sustainable resources such as fossil fuels for energy. As well as being a limited resource, the burning of fossil fuels also raises issues to do with pollution and climate change – the subject of the next chapter.

The fact the State of the World Population Report comes from the family planning sector of the UN suggests a continued emphasis on restricting population growth, especially in the 31 or so very economically poor countries with birth rates of five or more per woman and thus more than double the replacement level said to be 2.1 per woman. However the conundrum of the connection of a high fertility rate with poor levels of survival and poor longevity raises more questions about what exactly the policy, resources and education priorities should be.

Pope John Paul II acknowledged that there is a demographic problem but denounced systematic anti-childbearing campaigns which, on the basis of a distorted view of the demographic problem and in a climate of "absolute lack of respect for the freedom of choice of the parties involved", often subject them "to intolerable pressures ... in order to force them to submit to this new form of oppression".[291]

In 1991, on the 100th anniversary of the Catholic social teaching document, *Rerum Novarum,* he wrote:

> These criticisms are directed not so much against an eco-

---

290 UNFPA, *State of World Population report: People and Possibilities in a World of 7 Billion*, op. cit.
291 Pope John Paul II, *Sollicitudo Rei Socialis*, op. cit., n. 25.

nomic system as against an ethical and cultural system. The economy in fact is only one aspect and one dimension of the whole of human activity. If economic life is absolutized, if the production and consumption of goods become the centre of social life and society's only value, not subject to any other value, the reason is to be found not so much in the economic system itself as in the fact that the entire socio-cultural system, by ignoring the ethical and religious dimension, has been weakened, and ends by limiting itself to the production of goods and services alone.[292]

The question of overpopulation and the recognition that the earth has finite resources is raised as a concern for the future. The issue is changing as development of technology, changes in employment and attitudes to family formation and population policies have had effects. The problem now is different from what Reverend Malthus described in 1798, because food production has dramatically changed with the rise of factory farming. It is different again from what it was in 1973 when the Australian Bishops released a social justice statement on the population question.[293] Developed countries now have fertility rates below replacement level and that is bringing its own problem in relation to the ageing of the population. The developing countries have also dropped their rates so that many are close to replacement level or, like China, below it. Nevertheless the least developed countries have retained fertility rates of over five per woman.

The issue of population is a source of tension for the Church because the means used in international and government policy to reduce population growth is to advocate contraception and abortion under the heading of "reproductive health" and some countries have adopted coercive policies to limit family size. Both

---

[292] Pope John Paul II, *Centesimus Annus*, op. cit., n. 40.
[293] Australian Catholic Bishops Conference, 'Population in Perspective', Social Justice Statement, 1973.

overpopulation and the spread of sexually transmissible infection have become sticks with which to beat the Church, blaming the Church for its moral positions on contraception and abortion for hindering efforts to control poverty and disease.[294] The Church is accused of being irresponsible, anti-woman and interfering in strategies to prevent the spread of disease. However, the data would indicate otherwise – where the Church policies have had more influence the incidence of HIV/AIDS has been lower.[295]

There is also an internal issue for the Church with respect to the population question and the environment. The Church recognizes the need for use of natural resources to be sustainable and for good stewardship, as was discussed previously. What then should the attitude of the Church be to the population question? What should be the attitude of young couples engaged in family formation? Is there an ideal family size? If so, does that ideal family size relate to local issues such as our below replacement level birth-rate and the resultant ageing of our population and loss of workforce, or should it relate globally where the population is still growing at a rate that may see it double in the next 70 years? Is there a population problem at all? That is to say are there grounds for simply trusting that increases in food productivity, changes to more sustainable uses of resources and reduction of individual consumption will match population growth into the predictable future? Is the problem one of overconsumption, particularly by developed countries, rather than a population problem? In relation to population growth, the Church supports sustainable engagement with the environment, stewardship rather than exploitation, and responsible family planning by couples and government policies that are consistent

---

[294] The relative effect of Church policies on sexually transmissible infection is discussed in Volume IV of this About Bioethics series: *Motherhood, Embodied Love and Technology* (Connor Court 2013), chapter 15, "Prevention of Sexually Transmissible Infection: Was the Church wrong?" pp. 240ff.
[295] Ibid.

with their dignity. One question to ask is whether education reduces both population growth and poverty. The answers to that question have led to policies focussing on women's and children's health and education. Central to those approaches is how to ensure that policies and their implementation respect individual freedom, worth and dignity and bodily integrity.

2. Malthus

The population question is not new, the possibility that human beings might overpopulate was discussed by the ancients. Plato, for instance, thought that the City-State had an optimum number of about 60,000 with about 5,000 being citizens and the rest slaves and non-citizens. His reasoning was based on the numbers needed for defence and for the various forms of land use needed. His ideas for controlling population also included radical ideas for family life and eugenics with only some selected individuals being licensed to reproduce.[296]

The population question was presented scientifically in 1798 by the Reverend Thomas Malthus reflecting concerns at the time about the impact of the industrial revolution. Malthus was a Fellow of the Royal Society and an economist.

He began his analysis with two propositions: "First, that food is necessary to the existence of man. Secondly, that the passion between the sexes is necessary and will remain nearly in its present state."[297]

The central elements of his argument based on these two propositions may be summarized as in the following:

---
296 Plato, *The Republic*, ed. G.R.F. Ferrari, trans. T. Griffith, Cambridge, Cambridge University Press, 2000.
297 Thomas Robert Malthus, *An Essay on the Principle of Population*, New York, Dutton, 1960, p. 70.

> Population, when unchecked, increases in a geometrical ratio. Subsistence increases only in an arithmetical ratio. A slight acquaintance with numbers will shew the immensity of the first power in comparison to the second.
>
> By that law of our nature which makes food necessary to the life of man, the effects of these two unequal powers must be kept equal.
>
> This implies a strong and constantly operating check on population from the difficulty of subsistence. This difficulty must fall somewhere and must necessarily be severely felt by a large portion of mankind.[298]

His fear was that, with the shift towards an industrialized society away from subsistence, the natural checks on population growth by the limits on food supply had been overcome.

In contrast to other scholars at the time who predicted that industrialization would overcome the food shortages and that education would perfect humanity, he held that mankind will continue to reproduce until he consumes all available food supply, and then will only be prevented from expanding further by simple hunger. Therefore:

> The natural inequality of the two powers of population and of production in the earth, and that great law of our nature which must constantly keep their effects equal, form the great difficulty that to me appears insurmountable in the way to the perfectibility of society ... And it appears, therefore, to be decisive against the possible existence of a society, all the members of which should live in ease, happiness, and comparative leisure; and feel no anxiety about providing the means of subsistence for themselves and families.

Consequently, if the premises are just, the argument is

---
298 Ibid., p. 71.

conclusive against the perfectibility of the mass of mankind.[299]

In the second edition of his work but not in later editions, presumably because it provoked controversy, Malthus wrote:

> A man who is born into a world already possessed, if he cannot get subsistence from his parents on whom he has a just demand, and if the society do not want his labour, has no claim of right to the smallest portion of food, and, in fact, has no business to be where he is. At nature's mighty feast there is no vacant cover for him. She tells him to be gone, and will quickly execute her own orders, if he does not work upon the compassion of some of her guests. If these guests get up and make room for him, other intruders immediately appear demanding the same favour. The report of a provision for all that come, fills the hall with numerous claimants. The order and harmony of the feast is disturbed, the plenty that before reigned is changed into scarcity; and the happiness of the guests is destroyed by the spectacle of misery and dependence in every part of the hall, and by the clamorous importunity of those, who are justly enraged at not finding the provision which they had been taught to expect. The guests learn too late their error, in counter-acting those strict orders to all intruders, issued by the great mistress of the feast, who, wishing that all guests should have plenty, and knowing she could not provide for unlimited numbers, humanely refused to admit fresh comers when her table was already full.[300]

This sounds like today's Australian debate over immigration and the Government and Opposition claims that, despite their

---

299 Ibid., p. 72.
300 Garrett Hardin, 'The Feast of Malthus', *The Social Contract*, Spring 1998, http://www.thesocialcontract.com/cgi-bin/showarticle.pl?articleID=737 (accessed 1 September 2011).

Appendix A: The Population Question

legal right to seek asylum, if we do not punish and exclude people arriving on boats they will greatly increase. The logic has been so compellingly bi-partisan that the ordinary principles of law in relation to punishing the innocent, and the ordinary decency of providing succour and safe haven for someone fleeing persecution seems to have been overridden. Deterring people from risking themselves to the uncertainties of merciless people smugglers seems to know few bounds, including the punishment of innocent children.

Malthus, in Chapters 18 and 19 of his book, puts forward a theory on the problem of evil in which he argues that humankind is in its nature slothful and, without evil, would simply doze through the day. Evil in the form of discomforts such as cold, hunger and thirst, is needed to stir him from his sloth, to wake him up so that he is forced to exercise his intelligence.[301] These theodicy chapters were also dropped from the later editions.

In the 20th century, Malthusian economic views on population became not just an oddity but dominant in scientific thinking and were reflected in government policies in countries such as India and China and were linked to economic aid from developed countries to less developed countries. Paul Ehrlich was an example of someone with this view. In his book, *The Population Bomb*, he wrote:

> When he [Indian Minister Sripati Chandrasekhar] suggested sterilizing all Indian males with three or more children, we should have applied pressure on the Indian government to go ahead with the plan. We should have volunteered logistic support in the form of helicopters, vehicles, and surgical instruments. We should have sent doctors to aid in the program by setting up centers for training para-medical personnel to do vasectomies. Coer-

---
301 Malthus, op. cit., chapters 18-19.

cion? Perhaps, but coercion in a good cause. I am sometimes astounded at the attitudes of Americans who are horrified at the prospect of our government insisting on population control as the price of food aid. All too often the very same people are fully in support of applying military force against those who disagree with our form of government or our foreign policy. We must be relentless in pushing for population control around the world.[302]

Western governments, then and since, linked their aid to developing countries to the provision of contraception and abortion. Current United Nations policy, adopted by Australia and many other countries that provide aid, states:

> Efforts to slow population growth, reduce poverty, achieve economic progress, improve environmental protection and reduce unsustainable consumption and production patterns are mutually reinforcing. Sustained economic growth within the context of sustainable development is essential to eradicate poverty. Eradicating poverty will contribute to slowing population growth and to achieving early population stabilization. Women are generally the poorest of the poor. They are also key actors in the development process. Eliminating all forms of discrimination against women is thus a prerequisite for eradicating poverty, promoting sustained economic growth, ensuring quality family planning and reproductive health services, and achieving balance between population and available resources.
>
> Governments should invest in, promote, monitor and evaluate the education and skill development of women and girls and the legal and economic rights of women. They should do the same with all aspects of reproduc-

---

302 Paul R. Ehrlich, *The Population Bomb*, New York, Ballantine Books, 1968, pp. 165–166.

tive health, including family planning. The international community should continue to promote a supportive economic environment, particularly for developing countries and countries with economies in transition in their attempt to eradicate poverty and achieve sustained economic growth within the context of sustainable development.[303]

3. World Population Rates and Projections

Government policy is set against a background in which the world's population, now said to be seven billion, is growing at a pace of more than 90 million persons a year. The UN states that many of the resources on which future generations will depend are being depleted at alarming rates and pollution is intensifying, driven by wasteful consumption, the unprecedented growth in human numbers, persistent poverty, and social and economic inequality. While fertility has declined throughout the developing world since the 1970s to below replacement, the least developed countries (31 countries) have total fertility levels above five children per woman.[304]

The picture in more developed countries is the reverse with most having a birth rate well below replacement which is 2.1 children per woman. 107 (47%) of the world's 230 countries have a birth rate below replacement including the European countries which average 1.59, the United States 2.06, Australia 1.78, Canada 1.58, China 1.54 and New Zealand 2.09. The world fertility rate

---

303 UNFPA, *Programme of Action of the International Conference on Population and Development*, Cairo, 1994, summary retrieved from http://ngosbeyond2014.org/articles/2011/10/1/summary-of-the-programme-of-action.html (accessed 2010-2014).
304 UN Department of Social and Economic Affairs, 'What would it take to accelerate fertility decline in the least developed countries?', *UN Population Division Policy Brief*, March 2009, http://www.un.org/esa/population/publications/UNPD_policybriefs/UNPD_policy_brief1.pdf (accessed 1 September 2011).

is 2.56 children per women. 68 (30%) countries have a fertility rate greater than 3 per woman, leaving a further 55 (24%) with a rate only marginally higher than replacement.[305] The countries that have a high birth rate also have lower survival rates so it is hard to grasp the nature of the problem. Arguably, based on the evidence, as poverty reduces living standards will improve, as will longevity and education, and the economic pressure for large families to work the family farm will reduce resulting in lower birth rates.

In regard to absolute population growth rates it is worth considering that at a 4% growth rate a country's population will double in about 18 years; at a 1% growth rate it will take about 70 years. The average population growth rate for the world is 1.17%. Only 35 countries have a population growth rate of zero or less. The Holy See has a zero population growth rate and is not listed in the birth rate figures. Italy, Poland, Croatia, Germany, Japan, Hungary, Russia and the Baltic States all have negative growth. The growth rate of the US is 0.97, Australia 1.01 and the UK 0.48.[306] Given the below replacement birth rates it is clear that the population of the latter countries is growing as a result of immigration.

It is true that if the population were to continue to grow at the current rate then the population would double at least every 70 years. Presumably there is a finite limit to the size of the population that the world can continue to provide with food and water. If we keep doubling in size in that way then that point would at some time be reached.

This is on a world scale. Country by country the population

---

305 The World Factbook, *Country Comparison – Total Fertility Rate*, Central Intelligence Agency, Washington, 2009, https://www.cia.gov/library/publications/the-world-factbook/rankorder/2127rank.html (accessed 2010-2014).
306 UN Department of Economic and Social Affairs, Population Division (2007), 'Table A.8 – average annual rate of population change by country', *World Population Prospects: The 2006 Revision*, retrieved from http://www.un.org/esa/population/publications/wpp2006/WPP2006_Highlights_rev.pdf (accessed 2010-2014).

Appendix A: The Population Question

pressure on the environment may be greater or lesser, depending on the resources available. Clearly there is not an even availability of resources with some countries being very rich in resources and others much poorer.

There is a negative correlation between education standards and fertility rates. There is also a positive correlation between poverty and fertility rates and a negative correlation between fertility and survival rates or longevity. The better the survival chances, the fewer the children borne, which makes some sense. In countries that are better educated, people are wealthier, live longer and have fewer children.

This would suggest that if the world's governments were to overcome poverty and provide people with education the population growth would reduce. There is a chicken and egg problem in relation to whether poverty causes population growth or excess population causes poverty. But, as mentioned above, in many developing countries with high birth rates the standard of living has actually improved. The relationship between education and birth rates would suggest that poverty causes population pressures rather than the other way around. If you are poor, lack food and health care, and have a low expectation of survival it is likely to lead you to have more children, especially as poor countries tend to depend on subsistence farming which is very labour intensive.

From the 5.7 billion of 2009, the world's population is expected to cross 9 billion by 2050 and 10 billion by the turn of the century with the developing countries accounting for the bulk of the growth. Fertility rates are declining and this trend is expected to continue over the next fifty years causing the world population to eventually stabilize (probably between 8 and 12 billion), however the rate of decline is unknown. According to United Nations estimates, if the total fertility rate of almost every country reached 2.1 children per woman then the world population would be 9.4 billion by 2050. If worldwide fertility only declined to 2.6 children per woman then the world population in 2050 would be 11.2 billion (almost double that of 2009).[307]

4. Ageing of Developed Populations

An important matter to consider in any discussion of population numbers is the ageing of the population that has occurred in developed countries as a result of a rapid decline in the birth rate and increased longevity associated with higher standards of living and healthcare. The "ageing" of the population has been brought about by fact that the proportion above 65 years is increasing and the proportion below 15 years is decreasing. The following table[308] shows the change in terms of percentages:

Population as at 30 June (millions of people)

Age	1970	2010	2020	2030	2040	2050
0-14	3.8	4.2	4.9	5.4	5.7	6.2
15-64	7.9	15.0	16.6	18.2	20.0	21.6
65-84	1.0	2.6	3.7	4.8	5.6	6.3
85+	0.1	0.4	0.5	0.8	1.3	1.8
Total	12.5	22.2	25.7	29.2	32.6	35.9

Percentage of total population

0-14	28.8	19.1	19.0	18.3	17.4	17.2
15-64	62.8	67.4	64.7	62.4	61.3	60.2
65-84	7.8	11.7	14.3	16.8	17.2	17.6
85+	0.5	1.8	2.1	2.7	4.0	5.1

Note that from 1970 to 2010 the proportion under 15 dropped

---

[307] 'Countries Compared by People > Population growth rate', compiled by NationMaster, *CIA World Factbooks 2003-2013*, http://www.nationmaster.com/graph/peo_pop_gro_rat-people-population-growth-rate (accessed 2010-2014).

[308] '2010 Intergenerational Report Overview – Australia's Ageing Population', Australian Government: The Treasury, 2010, http://archive.treasury.gov.au/igr/igr2010/default.asp (accessed 2010-2014).

Appendix A: The Population Question

from 28.8% to 19.1% while the proportion above 65 went from 8.3% to 13.5%. That is a significant change. The lower birth rate and greater longevity would seem to be significant factors.

The Australian Treasury projects that the ageing of the population will have quite dramatic economic effects. The column graph below projects increases in the percentage of Gross Domestic Product needed for health care, age related pensions and aged care compared to other income support and spending on education and defence.[309]

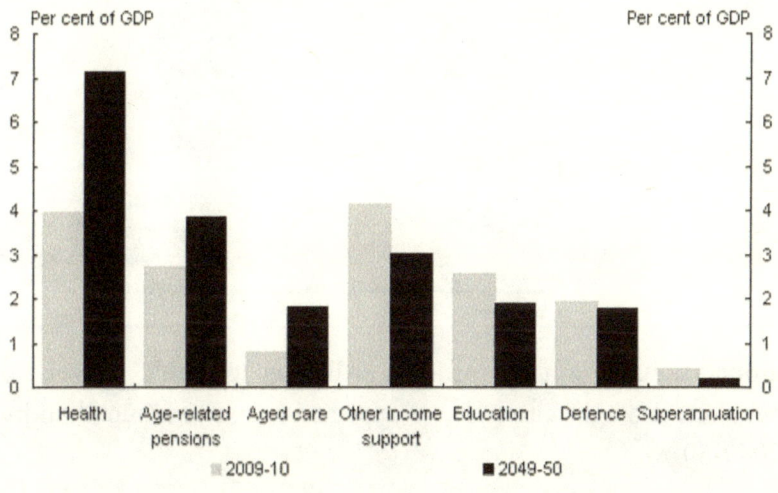

Treasury predicts that population ageing will increase spending on health, age-related pensions and aged care. Escalating health costs associated with technological advancements, such as new medicines, and increasing demand for higher quality services will add to fiscal pressures from ageing. At the same time, slowing economic growth as a result of an ageing population will reduce the capacity of Australia to fund this increasing spending. Today,

---

309 Ibid.

Faith, Science and the Environment

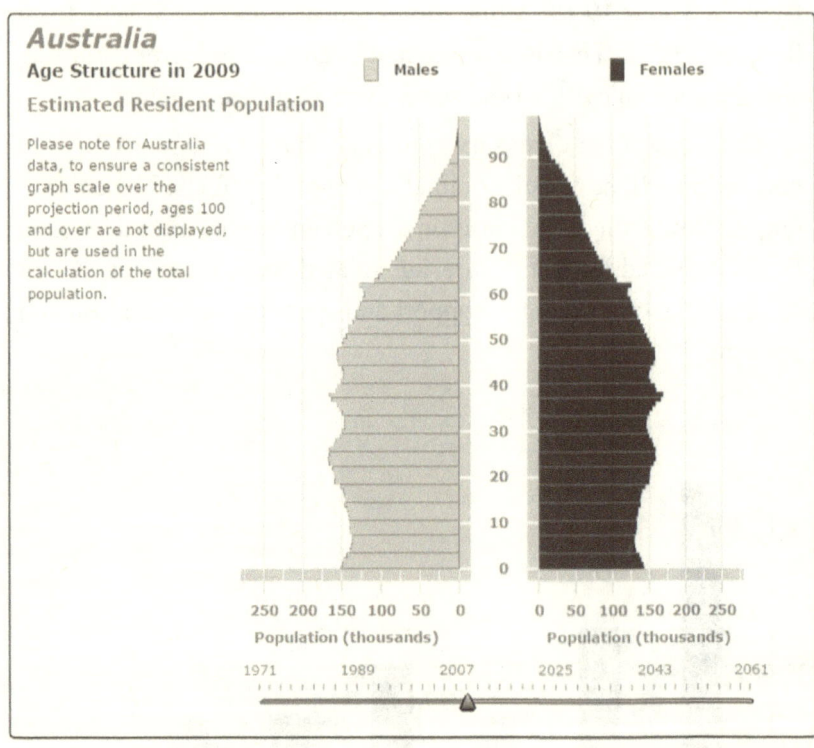

around a quarter of total spending is directed to health, age-related pensions and aged care. This is expected to rise to around half by 2049-50.[310]

The problem is a short term one: it reflects the fact that the baby boom after the Second World War followed by much lower birth rates for subsequent generations has created a significant disproportion between the larger cohort of baby boomers now becoming aged and the subsequent generations. Over time, balance can be expected to be restored when the baby boomer generations die off but, in the meantime, there will be significant pressure on subsequent generations to support those who have retired. That is

---

310 Ibid.

Appendix A: The Population Question

why Australian governments have made superannuation payments compulsory for salary earners and have created the Future Fund to invest current Government income to meet future aged care costs. On the previous page is the population pyramid for 2009[311] and below for comparison is the pyramid for 1911.[312] It is the population bulge of people now in midlife that will create the disproportion of aged people in the future, compared to 1911 when an even tapering of the population occurred as people aged.

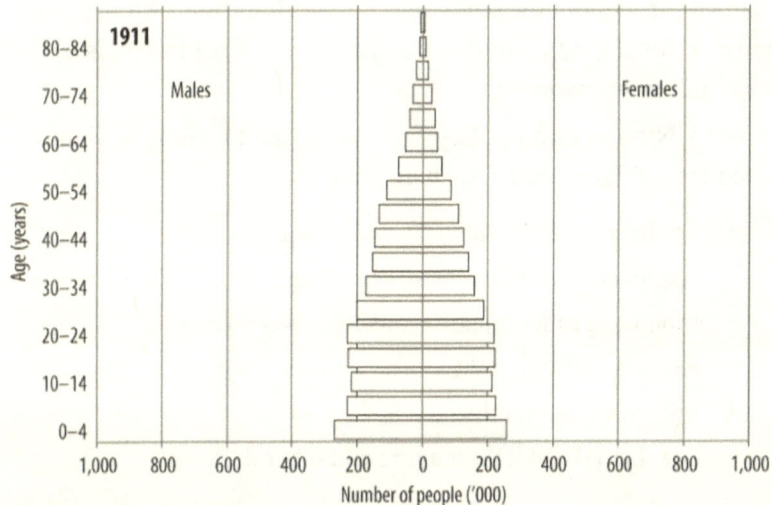

5. UN Population Policy

The United Nations draws a distinction between the developed nations, the developing nations and the least developed nations. The developing nations represent a "success" story for the UN policy with fertility rates declining, so that the average fertility rate in developing nations in 2009 was 2.8 per woman, well on

---

311 'Measures of Australia's Progress', Australian Bureau of Statistics, 2009, retrieved from http://betaworks.abs.gov.au/betaworks/betaworks.nsf/projects/MeasuresOfAustralia'sProgress/population/index.htm (accessed 2010-2014).
312 'Fertility and family policy in Australia', Australian Institute of Family Studies, Research Paper No. 41, 2008, https://aifs.gov.au/publications/fertility-and-family-policy-australia/2-fertility-rates-demographic-structure-and (accessed 2010-2014).

the way down to the desired target of replacement level of 2.1. It has occurred though at the price of an ageing population and the resultant prediction of labour shortage and growing demand for aged care. However, the least developed nations, of which there are 49, are considered to be a continuing problem for expanding the world population. The UN holds that high fertility rates hinder the reduction of poverty and the achievement of other internationally agreed development goals.[313] While fertility has declined throughout the developing world since the 1970s, most of the least developed countries still have total fertility levels above five children per woman.[314]

The UN population policy falls under the heading of what are called the Millennium Goals which are to:

- Eradicate extreme poverty and hunger.
- Achieve universal primary education.
- Promote gender equality and empower women.
- Reduce child mortality.
- Improve maternal health.
- Combat HIV/AIDS, malaria and other diseases.

Under the fifth goal, to improve maternal health, the target is to achieve, by 2015, universal access to reproductive health and the indicators for it are:

- Maternal mortality ratio.
- Proportion of births attended by skilled health personnel.

---

313 UN Economic and Social Council, 'World population monitoring, focusing on the contribution of the Programme of Action of the International Conference on Population and Development to the internationally agreed development goals, including the Millennium Development Goals – Report of the Secretary-General', Commission on Population and Development: Forty-second session, item 3 of the provisional agenda, 2009, [E/CN.9/2009/3], https://documents-dds-ny.un.org/doc/UNDOC/GEN/N09/212/29/PDF/N0921229.pdf?OpenElement (accessed 2010-2014).
314 UN Department of Social and Economic Affairs, op. cit.

- Contraceptive prevalence rate.
- Adolescent birth rate.
- Antenatal care coverage.
- Unmet need for family planning.

It is not difficult to see why the Vatican and the Church's teachings on contraception and abortion are considered an international problem for the United Nations.

The UN defines "reproductive health" as a state of complete physical, mental and social well-being, and not merely the absence of reproductive disease or infirmity. Reproductive health deals with the reproductive processes, functions and system at all stages of life. The International Conference on Population and Development Programme of Action states that:

> reproductive health ... implies that people are able to have a satisfying and safe sex life and that they have the capability to reproduce and the freedom to decide if, when and how often to do so. Implicit in this last condition are the right of men and women to be informed and to have access to safe, effective, affordable and acceptable methods of family planning of their choice, as well as other methods of their choice for regulation of fertility which are not against the law, and the right of access to appropriate health care services that will enable women to go safely through pregnancy and childbirth and provide couples with the best chance of having a healthy infant ... Reproductive health includes sexual health, the purpose of which is the enhancement of life and personal relations, and not merely counselling and care related to reproduction and sexually transmitted diseases.[315]

---

315 UN Population Division, 'Guidelines on Reproductive Health', Population Information Network (POPIN), http://www.un.org/popin/unfpa/taskforce/guide/iatfreph.gdl.html (accessed 2010-2014).

The least developed countries as a group and in their majority are lagging behind in the transition to low fertility and have rapidly growing populations. In 2009 the UN Population Division concluded that:

- Lack of access to family planning and, in particular, to modern methods of contraception is a major cause of the persistence of high fertility as indicated by the high levels of unmet need for family planning prevalent in most least developed countries having the requisite data.
- Expansion of access to family planning requires government commitment and effective action to disseminate information about contraceptive methods and the benefits of smaller families.
- Strengthening and expanding family planning services requires adequate funding and access to supplies. Increases in donor funding for family planning would make a major contribution in this regard given that, since the mid-1990s, most least developed countries have experienced a per capita decrease in donor funding for family planning.
- Investments in family planning are cost effective because of the strong synergistic effects of longer inter-birth intervals and lower fertility with other development goals. For every dollar spent in family planning, between 2 and 6 dollars can be saved in interventions aimed at achieving other development goals.[316]

But this treats the issue as one of information and supply of family planning methods only rather than motivation, and the effects of standards of living on longevity, and the desire to have larger families for labour purposes in subsistence farming – an

---
316 UN Department of Social and Economic Affairs, op. cit.

approach that also seems to be a male preference to the detriment of girls and women and their survival. As we have seen, the issue of motivation is more complex, with better health and standards of living associated with reduced birth rates. Knowledge and supply of methods of family planning are significant but there are other factors related to treating the causes of ill-health and mortality that would seem to be important. Lifting standards of living would seem to be a priority and, as the evidence shows, this can be done without first having to reduce population growth. Rather, with greater longevity and higher standards of living, the motivation for larger families diminishes.

6. The Catholic Church and UN Population Policy

In 2010, the UN supported a *Reproductive Health Bill* in the Philippines. At the time, according to the University of the Philippines:

> ... the Philippines has the highest fertility rate in Southeast Asia at 3.3 percent, followed by Cambodia 3 percent, Malaysia 2.5 percent, and Vietnam 2.1 percent. The Philippines also has the highest population growth rate at 2 percent and is the second most populous country in the region - behind Indonesia – with 92 million people.[317]

The bill mandates the government to "promote, without bias, all effective natural and modern methods of family planning that are medically safe and legal." Although abortion is recognized as illegal and punishable by law, the bill states that "the government shall ensure that all women needing care for post-abortion complications shall be treated and counseled in a humane, non-judgmental and compassionate manner." The bill calls for a "multi-

---

317 Integrated Regional Information Networks (IRIN), *Philippines: Battle over reproductive health bill intensifies*, 17 November 2010, http://www.refworld.org/docid/4ce6834c17.html (accessed 2010-2014).

dimensional approach" that integrates a component of family planning and responsible parenthood into all government anti-poverty programs. Under the bill, age-appropriate reproductive health and sexuality education is required from grade five to fourth year high school using "life-skills and other approaches."[318]

The Catholic Bishops Conference of the Philippines dismissed population growth as grounds for a new law:

> The population is not a problem. We are of the firm conviction that there is no need to legislate a national law on birth control. What the poor people need [from the government] is not contraception, but employment and economic opportunities.[319]

The tension between the teaching of the Catholic Church and the United Nations and secular government policy is obvious. But a distinction can usefully be made between the issue of whether population should be controlled or at least the rate of population growth reduced, on the one hand, and, on the other, how a reduction in population growth might be achieved. The teaching of the Church is clear in relation to the latter in that the Church rejects contraception and abortion. The position of the Church in relation to the issue of population growth is not so clear. The Church is clear that human beings should be the subject of economic policy and not its object. In other words, improvements in the economy should only be sought in order to improve conditions for human beings. The economy is never more important than human beings. On a trip to Madrid for World Youth Day, Pope Benedict observed, "The economy cannot function as a self-regulated econ-

---

318 Philippine Senate and House of Representatives, RH Bill – Philippines: full text of reproductive health and related measures, May 2010, http://www.likhaan.org/content/rh-bill-philippines-full-text-reproductive-health-and-related-measures (accessed 2010-2014).
319 IRIN, op. cit.

omy. Man must be at the economy's centre, which is not profit but solidarity."[320]

In *Caritas in Veritate* he made a more complicated but related claim:

> It should be remembered that the reduction of cultures to the technological dimension, even if it favours short-term profits, in the long term impedes reciprocal enrichment and the dynamics of cooperation. It is important to distinguish between short- and long-term economic or sociological considerations. Lowering the level of protection accorded to the rights of workers, or abandoning mechanisms of wealth redistribution in order to increase the country's international competitiveness, hinder the achievement of lasting development. Moreover, the human consequences of current tendencies towards a short-term economy – sometimes very short-term – need to be carefully evaluated. This requires *further and deeper reflection on the meaning of the economy and its goals*, as well as a profound and far-sighted revision of the current model of development, so as to correct its dysfunctions and deviations. This is demanded, in any case, by the earth's state of ecological health; above all it is required by the cultural and moral crisis of man, the symptoms of which have been evident for some time all over the world.[321]

However, it would seem to be consistent with that view that one could envisage that there is a reasonable limit to the population that can be sustained by the world's resources and that population growth should be responsible. What the sustainable population

---

[320] 'Pope arrives in Spain saying economy not just for profit', *The Australian*, 18 August 2011, http://www.theaustralian.com.au/news/world/pope-arrives-in-spain-saying-economy-not-just-for-profit/story-e6frg6so-1226117727570 (accessed 22 September 2011).

[321] Pope Benedict XVI, *Caritas in Veritate*, op. cit., n. 32.

limit of the earth is, however, is clearly affected by rates of consumption of resources and whether the uses of resources are sustainable. The more we consume and the more we consume in an unsustainable way, the greater the pressure on the issue of population. That suggests that we have very strong obligations in relation to consumption and sustainability.

The Catholic Church is often accused of causing poverty and the spread of infectious disease because it refuses to advocate contraception and teaches that it is immoral. That linked also with the issue of abortion leads to claims that the Church is at least irresponsible. Some have even accused the Church of being responsible for loss of life by hindering the prevention of HIV/AIDS and other sexually transmissible infections.

Pope Benedict rejects the claim that population growth is the cause of poverty. In his Peace Day Message of 2009 he wrote:

> Poverty is often considered a consequence of demographic change. For this reason, there are international campaigns afoot to reduce birth-rates, sometimes using methods that respect neither the dignity of the woman, nor the right of parents to choose responsibly how many children to have; graver still, these methods often fail to respect even the right to life. The extermination of millions of unborn children, in the name of the fight against poverty, actually constitutes the destruction of the poorest of all human beings. And yet it remains the case that in 1981, around 40% of the world's population was below the threshold of absolute poverty, while today that percentage has been reduced by as much as a half, and whole peoples have escaped from poverty despite experiencing substantial demographic growth. This goes to show that resources to solve the problem of poverty do exist, even in the face of an increasing population. Nor must it be forgotten

Appendix A: The Population Question

that, since the end of the Second World War, the world's population has grown by four billion, largely because of certain countries that have recently emerged on the international scene as new economic powers, and have experienced rapid development specifically because of the large number of their inhabitants. Moreover, among the most developed nations, those with higher birth-rates enjoy better opportunities for development. In other words, population is proving to be an asset, not a factor that contributes to poverty.[322]

One of the factors involved in this debate going back at least as far as Plato and Aristotle is whether human population is seen as an economic asset. The simple equation that predicts eventual food shortage as a result of population tends to ignore productivity improvements. Where food shortages currently exist they seem to be a result of political unrest and consequent loss of productivity rather than reflecting population growth. The terrible circumstances in Africa where some countries experience famine are testimony to the effects of political instability. The "greening of India" was not brought about by decreasing the population, but by relative political stability and better management of agriculture.

That is not to deny that there is a limit to the capacity of the Earth's resources and that there must therefore be a limit to its productivity and hence a limit to the population that can be fed. The question would seem to be about what size population can be sustained by improving the productivity of the land in a sustainable way.

The reality is that the rate of population growth is significantly declining so the issue is whether it will reach a stage of zero

---

[322] Pope Benedict XVI, *Fighting Poverty To Build Peace*, 1 January 2009, n. 3, http://www.vatican.va/holy_father/benedict_xvi/messages/peace/documents/hf_ben-xvi_mes_20081208_xlii-world-day-peace_en.html (accessed 2010-2014).

growth within the absolute limit of productivity. We would seem to be a long way from the absolute limit, but precisely what that limit may be is an empirical matter about which we do not have knowledge of all the factors. In the time of Malthus they could not have predicted the developments in technology and science that have so improved productivity. The growth of knowledge is not predictable. The comparison between projected population levels and projected productivity has too many uncertain variables to be accurate.

The factors that influence rates of population growth are also difficult to assess both in the present and even more so for the future. Where governments have sought to intervene by imposing economic penalties for exceeding an imposed birth rate, it has been at enormous cost to individual freedom and wellbeing and resulted in population ageing and resultant loss of the proportion of people in the productive workforce.

The policies, mentioned earlier, of linking aid to developing countries to the provision of family planning services and abortion, so-called "reproductive health", raise questions about cultural hegemony and intolerance, with the developed world thinking that it has a mission to evangelize the less and least developed countries with its ideas about abortion and contraception as necessary agents for population control.

Pope Benedict addressed the priorities in relation to population policy again in *Caritas in Veritate*:

> The notion of rights and duties in development must also take account of the problems associated with *population growth*. This is a very important aspect of authentic development, since it concerns the inalienable values of life and the family. To consider population increase as the primary cause of underdevelopment is mistaken, even from an economic point of view. Suffice it to consider, on the

one hand, the significant reduction in infant mortality and the rise in average life expectancy found in economically developed countries, and on the other hand, the signs of crisis observable in societies that are registering an alarming decline in their birth rate. Due attention must obviously be given to responsible procreation, which among other things has a positive contribution to make to integral human development. The Church, in her concern for man's authentic development, urges him to have full respect for human values in the exercise of his sexuality. It cannot be reduced merely to pleasure or entertainment, nor can sex education be reduced to technical instruction aimed solely at protecting the interested parties from possible disease or the "risk" of procreation. This would be to impoverish and disregard the deeper meaning of sexuality, a meaning which needs to be acknowledged and responsibly appropriated not only by individuals but also by the community. It is irresponsible to view sexuality merely as a source of pleasure, and likewise to regulate it through strategies of mandatory birth control. In either case materialistic ideas and policies are at work, and individuals are ultimately subjected to various forms of violence. Against such policies, there is a need to defend the primary competence of the family in the area of sexuality, as opposed to the State and its restrictive policies, and to ensure that parents are suitably prepared to undertake their responsibilities.[323]

7. Governments and Population Policy

The Governments of China and India have both had population policies designed to reduce population growth and the policies have been successful. According to the World Bank, China's birth

---

323 Pope Benedict XVI, *Caritas in Veritate*, op. cit., n. 44.

rate peaked in 1964 at six children per women and by 2009 had fallen to 1.7, less than replacement level and is now 1.5. In India the birth rate dropped from 5.9 in 1960 to 2.68 births per women in 2009.[324]

The other major factor in population growth is life expectancy. In China, in 1950, the life expectancy was 42 years for women and 39 for men. By 1998 it had risen to 71 for women and 68 for men.[325] In 2011, the estimated life expectancy was 76.94 years for women and 72.68 years for men.[326]

It is significant that as the life expectancy rose the birth rate dropped. This would make sense from the point of view of individual families even without government intervention. If more children survive child birth then the life expectancy will increase and as that happens then it would be expected that families would be less inclined to have as many children.

However, the changes in population growth in China were not entirely due to such natural causes. China's one child policy was established by Chinese leader Deng Xiaoping in 1979 to limit China's population growth. Although designated a "temporary measure," it continues a quarter-century after its establishment.[327] The policy limits couples to one child. Fines, pressures to abort a pregnancy, and even forced sterilization accompanied second or subsequent pregnancies. It is not an all-encompassing rule because

---

324 World Bank statistics, 'Fertility rate, total (births per woman)', 2011, http://data.worldbank.org/indicator/SP.DYN.TFRT.IN?cid=GPD_11 (accessed 26 September 2011).

325 'Issues and Trends in China's Demographic History', *Asia for Educators*, Columbia University, 2009, http://afe.easia.columbia.edu/special/china_1950_population.htm (accessed 26 September 2011).

326 CIA World Factbook, 'China life expectancy at birth', 2011, retrieved from http://www.indexmundi.com/china/life_expectancy_at_birth.html (accessed 26 September 2011).

327 Editor's note: The one child policy in China was revised in 2015 and is being formally phased out.

Appendix A: The Population Question

it has always been restricted to ethnic Han Chinese living in urban areas. Citizens living in rural areas and minorities living in China are not subject to the law. However, the rule has been estimated to have reduced population growth in the country of 1.3 billion by as much as 300 million people over its first twenty years.[328]

As published in The BMJ:

> Government family planning services became available as a contribution to maternal and child health in China from 1953. As the result of falling death rates, the population growth rate rose to 2.8%, leading to some 250 million additional people by 1970. After a century of rebellions, wars, epidemics, and the collapse of imperial authority, during which the annual population growth was probably no more than 0.3%, such an expansion was initially seen as part of China's new strength. Mao Zedong quoted a traditional saying: "Of all things in the world, people are the most precious."
>
> Rapid growth, however, put considerable strain on the government's efforts to meet the needs of its people. The fourth five year plan in 1970 included, for the first time, targets for population growth rate. Contraceptive and abortion services were extended into the rural areas, and there was extensive promotion of later marriage, longer intervals between births, and smaller families.
>
> Within five years the population growth rate fell to around 1.8%, and the target set for 1980 was a growth rate of 1%. To achieve this, each administrative unit introduced its own target and discussed and, when necessary, attempted to modify its population's fertility behaviour. At a local level, collective incomes and allocation of funds – for health care, welfare, and schools, for example – made it possible

---

[328] Matt Rosenberg, 'China's One Child Policy', *About Education*, http://geography.about.com/od/populationgeography/a/onechild.htm (accessed 26 September 2011).

for couples to understand the effect of their personal family choices on the community. They also made it possible for the community to exercise pressure on those who wished to have children outside the agreed plans.[329]

The implementation of the one child policy varied from province to province in the hands of local officials. Discouragement of larger families included financial levies on each additional child and sanctions which ranged from social pressure to curtailed career prospects for those in government jobs.[330]

China's population pyramid[331] in 1990 showed the severe effects of government policy and totalitarian rule:

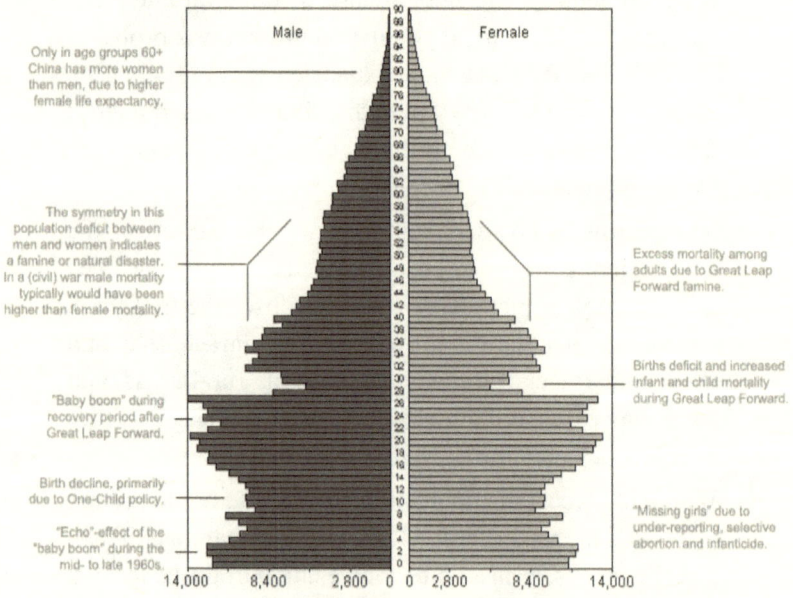

---

329 Penny Kane and Ching Y. Choi, 'China's one child family policy', *BMJ*, 9 Oct 1999, http://www.ncbi.nlm.nih.gov/pmc/articles/PMC1116810/ (accessed 2010-2014).
330 G. Feng and L. Hao, 'A summary of family planning regulations for 28 regions in China' [in Chinese], *Population Research*, 4, 1992, pp. 28-33.
331 National Bureau of Statistics of China, *China's population by age and sex in 1990* (based on 1990 population census), 1992, retrieved from http://www.china-profile.com/data/fig_p_19a_m.htm (accessed 2010-2014).

Appendix A: The Population Question

Time Magazine reported continued forced abortions and sterilization in 2007 claiming:

> Despite the growing consensus calling for change, however, Beijing continues to make enforcement of the policy one of the two main yardsticks by which the performance of local bureaucrats – and hence their prospects for advancement – are judged. (The other is tax collection.) It is this pressure from above to comply with population quotas that prompts local officials to adopt measures such as forced abortion (sometimes heart-rendingly late in term), forced sterilization and the like, says Nicolas Becquelin of New York-based Human Rights in China.[332]

One of the effects of limiting population is the gender specific impacts. If people are limited to having one child then in China it appears they would prefer that one child to be a boy. Female infanticide was a cultural practice in China historically but had declined after the communist revolution until the advent of new population policies. As published on the Gendercide Watch website:

> According to Zeng *et al.*, "The practice was largely forsaken in the 1950s, 1960s, and 1970s." (Zeng *et al.*, "Causes and Implications," p. 294.) Coale and Banister likewise acknowledge a "decline of excess female mortality after the establishment of the People's Republic ... assisted by the action of a strong government, which tried to modify this custom as well as other traditional practices that it viewed as harmful." (Coale and Banister, "Five Decades," p. 472.) But the number of "missing" women showed a sharp upward trend in the 1980s, linked by almost all scholars to the "one-child policy" introduced

---

[332] Simon Elegant, 'Why Forced Abortions Persist in China', *Time Magazine*, 30 April 2007.

by the Chinese government in 1979 to control spiralling population growth. Couples are penalized by wage-cuts and reduced access to social services when children are born "outside the plan." Johansson and Nygren found that while "sex ratios [were] generally within or fairly near the expected range of 105 to 106 boys per 100 girls for live births within the plan ... they are, in contrast, clearly far above normal for children born outside the plan, even as high as 115 to 118 for 1984-87. That the phenomenon of missing girls in China in the 1980s is related to the government's population policy is thus conclusively shown." (Sten Johansson and Ola Nygren, "The Missing Girls of China: A New Demographic Account," *Population and Development Review*, 17: 1 [March 1991], pp. 40-41.)[333]

The effect of the one child policy over four decades has created a gender imbalance in China. It is claimed that China now has 32 million more males than females under the age of 20.[334] The Chinese Academy of Social Sciences reports that for every 100 girls born in China, 119 boys are born.[335]

The tradition of a preference for sons was mainly responsible for China's high birth rate in the past, when large family size was normal and access to contraception and sex selective measures was limited. The one child policy was introduced to bring the high rate of population growth under control through fostering a culture of voluntarily having a small family. However, the policy itself is only partially responsible for the reduction in the total fertility rate. From the 1970s, before the policy was imposed, China saw

---

333 'Case Study: Female Infanticide', *Gendercide Watch*, http://www.gendercide.org/case_infanticide.html (accessed 26 September 2011).
334 T. Schure, 'China's Gender Imbalance', *Worldpress*, 6 January 2011, http://www.worldpress.org/Asia/3676.cfm#down (accessed 26 September 2011).
335 'China faces growing gender imbalance', *BBC News*, 11 January 2010, http://news.bbc.co.uk/2/hi/8451289.stm (accessed 26 September 2011).

an emerging culture of having a small family as a result of social and economic developments.[336]

The most dramatic decrease in the fertility rate, from 5.9 to 2.9, occurred between 1970 and 1979.[337] After the one child policy was introduced in 1979, the rate fell more gradually, and after 1995 it stabilized at around 1.7.[338] It has therefore been suggested that China's total fertility rate would have decreased even without the one child policy.[339] This large reduction in the fertility rate, whether by choice or by coercion, has inevitably increased the male to female ratio because of the preference for sons and the availability of contraception and sex selective measures. These changes in the sex ratio would probably have occurred even without the one child policy, but their effects would probably have been less serious.[340] This idea is supported by neighbouring countries in East Asia, which have no restriction on family size but have the same preference for sons as China; these countries have some of the lowest total fertility rates in the world but also have extremely high ratios of boys to girls at birth.[341]

Since 1952, India has worked to control its population growth. In 1983, the goal of the country's National Health Policy was to have a replacement value total fertility rate of 2.1 by the year

---

336 T. Liu and X. Zhang, 'Ratio of males to females in China', *BMJ*, 9 April 2009, http://dx.doi.org/10.1136/bmj.b483 (accessed 2010-2014).
337 T. Hesketh and W.X. Zhu, 'The one child family policy: the good, the bad, and the ugly', *BMJ*, 7 June 1997, http://www.ncbi.nlm.nih.gov/pmc/articles/PMC2126838/ (accessed 2010-2014).
338 J.Y. Wang, 'Evaluation of the fertility of Chinese women during 1990-2000', *Theses collection of 2001 national family planning and reproductive health survey*, Beijing, China Population Publishing House, 2003.
339 T. Hesketh, L. Lu and Z.W. Xing, 'The effect of China's one-child family policy after 25 years', *New England Journal of Medicine*, 15 September 2005.
340 Q.J. Ding and T. Hesketh, 'Family size, fertility preferences, and sex ratio in China in the era of the one child family policy: results from national family planning and reproductive health survey', *BMJ*, 11 May 2006.
341 Hesketh et al., op. cit.

2000. That did not occur. In 2000, the country established a new National Population Policy to stem the growth of the country's population. One of the primary goals of the policy was to reduce the total fertility rate to 2.1 by 2010. One of the steps along the path toward the goal in 2010 was a total fertility rate of 2.6 by 2002.[342]

Like China, one of the effects of efforts to curb population growth in India has been abortion and infanticide of female children. In 1999, His Excellency Mr. Dalit Ezhilmalai, Union Minister of State for Health and Family Welfare, Republic of India, made the following statement to the UN:

> We in India have initiated concerted efforts in one of the most important areas namely, advocating for the **protection of the girl child.** The increasing evidence of female foeticide and female infanticide, has lead the Government of India to adopt the National Plan of Action for the Girl Child (1991-2000) which also had been the force behind the enactment of the legislation to ban sex determination to prevent female foeticide. In India the **gender ideology,** where traditionally women's primary role is considered as mothers and housewives, is gradually undergoing a change and noteworthy enhancement has been achieved in women's education and participation in the work force thereby increasingly assuming the role as economic partner. In view of the Country's commitment towards implementation of the ICPD POA, during the current **Five Year Development Plan** (1997-2002) under implementation by Government of India concerted efforts are being made towards empowerment of women by creating enabling environment with requisite policies and

---

[342] Matt Rosenberg, 'India's Population: India Likely to Surpass China In Population by 2030', *About Education*, http://geography.about.com/od/obtainpopulationdata/a/indiapopulation.htm (accessed 26 September 2011).

programmes as well as legislative support. The Plan itself had the benefit of inputs from representatives of women thus setting up a participatory planning process by women themselves and making the plan gender responsive. **A draft National Policy for the Empowerment of Women** has been evolved in 1996 which focuses on changing societal attitudes to women and calls for efforts to eliminate gender based discrimination for promoting women's empowerment. We are also making efforts to promote women's **participation in the political process** by initiating efforts for getting parliamentary approval for reservation of the seats in the Parliament.[343]

In India, infanticide of female children is an age old phenomenon. However the practice of prenatal diagnosis and selected abortion has been a modern addition.

> In Jaipur, capital of the western state of Rajasthan, prenatal sex determination tests result in an estimated 3,500 abortions of female fetuses annually, according to a medical-college study. (Dahlburg, "Where killing baby girls 'is no big sin'.") Most strikingly, according to UNICEF, "A report from Bombay in 1984 on abortions after prenatal sex determination stated that 7,999 out of 8,000 of the aborted fetuses were females. Sex determination has become a lucrative business." (Zeng Yi *et al.*, "Causes and Implications of the Recent Increase in the Reported Sex Ratio at Birth in China," *Population and Development Review*, 19: 2 [June 1993], p. 297.)[344]

According to the UN, the gender ratio of male to female in

---

[343] Dalit Ezhilmalai (Union Minister for Health and Family Welfare, Republic of India), statement at The Hague Forum On Review of Progress in the Implementation of the ICPD Programme-of Action, 9 February 1999, retrieved from http://www.un.org/popin/icpd/icpd5/hague/india.pdf (accessed 26 September 2011).
[344] 'Case Study: Female Infanticide', *Gendercide Watch*, op. cit.

India has risen from 101 males to 100 females in 1951 to 107 males to 100 females in 2001. The reason for this dramatic shift is attributed by the UN to the introduction into India of methods of prenatal sex determination, such as amniocentesis and ultrasound technology. Some years earlier, India had also established a new and rather liberal law on abortion, which in many cases rendered the termination of a pregnancy considerably easier, for reasons ranging from foetal physical defect to contraception failure. As such, the change in abortion regulations was an offshoot of a government endeavour unrelated to sex discrimination.[345]

The law was primarily meant to address the issue of unwanted pregnancies, as part of a comprehensive family-planning strategy that encompassed many contraceptive options as well. But the combination of new technologies for pre-natal sex determination and abortion proved to be a dramatic cocktail which would quickly become an efficient sex-selection device. From the 1980s, sex-selective abortions became the primary method used to alter the sex composition of children.[346]

It is said that China and India could learn much from their neighbouring countries about reversing the worsening sex ratio. Korea was the first country to report very high male to female ratios at birth because of the preference for sons and the widespread use of sex selective technology. In 1992, the male to female ratio for fourth births in South Korea was an astounding 229:100, in sharp contrast to the overall ratio of 114:100. From the mid-1990s, however, a public awareness campaign warning of the dangers of such distortion, combined with strictly enforced laws forbidding

---

[345] Christophe Z. Guilmoto, 'Characteristics of Sex Ratio Imbalance in India, and Future Scenarios', 4th Asia Pacific Conference on Reproductive and Sexual health and Rights, UNFPA, Hyderabad, India, 29-31 October 2007, http://www.unfpa.org/gender/docs/studies/india.pdf (accessed 26 September 2011).
[346] M. Das Gupta and P.N. M. Bhat, 'Fertility decline and increased manifestation of sex bias in India', *Population Studies*, vol. 51, 1997, pp. 307-315.

sex selection technology, has led to a decline in the male to female ratio from 116:100 in 1998 to 110:100 in 2004.[347]

The problem of gender imbalance exists in China and India but it seems to be more of a cultural problem than a direct result of government policy. Government policy, especially in the case of China, put economic and coercive pressure on restricting the number of children, however the choice to favour one gender over the other, and to choose a male child, was not driven by government policy but has cultural causes in discriminatory attitudes in relation to employment and property ownership. In India, there is also the dowry system that makes a girl child a liability for the family in having to provide a dowry when she marries.

It is true that a small minority of countries have birth rates greater than five per woman, however the growth rate is trending downwards sharply. It is also the case that those countries that have high birth rates also have low average life expectancy. There does seem to be an association between increasing standards of health and life expectancy and lower birth rates. A significant part of the world population increase is due to increased life expectancy. The combination of reduced fertility and increased life expectancy has brought about the problem of ageing populations.

In that respect it is worth noting that the dramatic effect of China's population policies over the past forty years has created a significant difference between China, on the one hand, and India, on the other, where the population policies were not as draconian or effective as China's. China and India are sometimes cast in a long-term contest for global economic ascendancy even though China's economy, the world's second biggest, is four times the size of India's and its gross domestic product per capita is three

---

[347] C.B. Park and N.H. Cho, 'Consequences of son preference in a low fertility society: imbalance of the sex ratio at birth in Korea', *Population and Development Review*, vol. 21, no. 1, March 1995, pp. 59-84.

times higher (at market exchange rates). There is however a major difference: in China, years of stellar economic performance have been supported by the "demographic dividend" of a huge and expanding workforce of earlier high birth rates, followed by a dramatically reduced birth rate and a dramatically increased survival rate and longevity. This created a high proportion of the population at working age. The working-age population nearly doubled from 407 million in 1978 to 786 million in 2004, adding about 2 percentage points a year to GDP growth.[348]

However that advantage will start to fade, in 2015, when China's working-age population is forecast to peak and then start to decline. That will be the result of rising life expectancy and a falling fertility rate. As we have seen, in 1949 life expectancy in China was just 35 years, but now it is 75 and the birth rate has decreased to well below replacement. As a result, the proportion of elderly people to working age people will quadruple between now and 2050. United Nations projections suggest that by mid-century the proportion of the population aged over 60 will be 10 percentage points higher than the global average. The speed of China's demographic shift is illustrated by the ratio of children to over 60s – in 1975 there were six but by 2035 there will be just one or two.[349]

Japan, South Korea, Thailand and Singapore have a similar problem of an ageing population due to low birth rates and increased life expectancy. However the picture in India is quite different. With about 600 million people aged 25 or less, India's demographic dividend is far from over. About one million Indians are entering the workforce every month and that is expected to

---

348 Matt Wade, 'Youthful India may reap age dividend', *The Age*, 27 September 2011, retrieved from http://www.theage.com.au/business/youthful-india-may-reap-age-dividend-20110926-1kto9.html#ixzz1Z7oJTMpI (accessed 2010-2014).
349 Ibid.

Appendix A: The Population Question

continue for another two decades. The World Bank predicts India, along with Pakistan, the Philippines and Malaysia, will reap a demographic dividend for at least two more decades, while most economies grapple with ageing populations. The flood of new labour means India's ratio of elderly people to workers will be half that of China's by mid-century.[350]

One is left to wonder whether governments would have been well advised to stay out of the question of family size. High birth rates were associated with low life expectancy; it would seem likely that the birth rate would have adjusted itself when infant mortality dropped and life expectancy increased. It is likely that people would have adjusted family size as increased life expectancy altered the demographics of families. By interfering, governments would seem to have contributed to the ageing problem by artificially lowering the birth rate.

A major factor in dealing with the population question is the provision of better health and education. As economies move away from subsistence, the need to have children in order to work the land diminishes and people become involved in other pursuits that do not require manual labour. The emphasis on needing sons also seems to diminish. Rather than seeking to control population growth, governments would be better advised to look after the populations they have by ensuring that there is food, water, shelter, heath care and education. It is ironic that many countries now are trying to encourage people to have children after decades of beating the drum of a population explosion.

8. Responsible Family Planning

At some stage, in developed countries at least, most married couples address the question as to what size their family should be.

---

350 Ibid.

The evidence suggests that, if economic pressures are put to one side, most would prefer to have three or four children. A 2011 poll conducted by the 'Baby Center' website has the following result:[351]

If money, time, or resources weren't an issue, how many children would you like to have?

4%	One
24%	Two
33%	**Three**
26%	Four
14%	Five or more

That would seem to fit with most contemporary studies of the issue. However, if the resources factor is not excluded then the ideal number of children drops to two rather than three or four. The ideal family size is also affected by religious belief. A Gallup Poll in the US produced the following result (see next page):[352]

Today, Americans under age 35 appear to have a preference for larger families. 44% of those between the ages of 18 and 34 say that a family of three or more children is ideal, compared with 29% of those aged 35 to 54, and 33% of those 55 and older.[353]

In my parents' generation, large families were encouraged by the Church. I came from a family of eleven and amongst my cousins are several families of seven. However, in recent times the Church has been more reticent about addressing the issue of family size, except for maintaining that the dominant concern should not be materialism.

---

351 Poll conducted by Baby Center, 'How many children do you want?', http://www.babycenter.com.au/o4190/how-many-children-do-you-want (accessed 2010-2014).
352 J. Carroll, 'Americans: 2.5 Children Is "Ideal" Family Size', 26 June 2007, http://www.gallup.com/poll/27973/americans-25-children-ideal-family-size.aspx (accessed 27 September 2011).
353 Ibid.

Appendix A: The Population Question

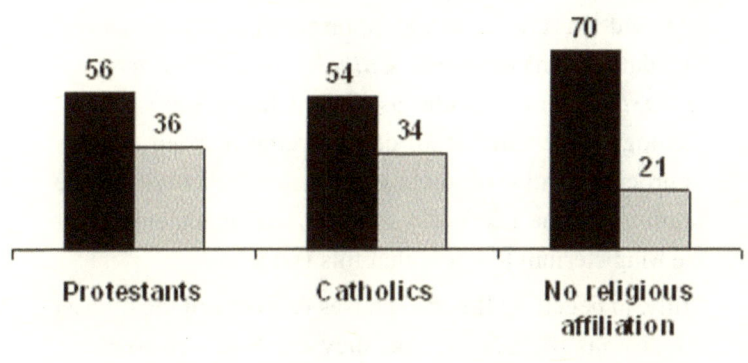

June 11-14, 2007

Pope John Paul II has noted:

> To maintain a joyful family requires much from both the parents and the children. Each member of the family has to become, in a special way, the servant of the others and share their burdens (cf. *Gal* 6:2; *Phil* 2:2). Each one must show concern, not only for his or her own life, but also for the lives of the other members of the family: their needs, their hopes, their ideals. Decisions about the number of children and the sacrifices to be made for them must not be taken only with a view to adding to comfort and preserving a peaceful existence. Reflecting upon this matter before God, with the graces drawn from the Sacrament, and guided by the teaching of the Church, parents will remind themselves that it is certainly less serious to deny their children certain comforts or material advantages than to deprive them of the presence of brothers and sisters, who

could help them to grow in humanity and to realize the beauty of life at all its ages and in all its variety.[354]

Pope John Paul II also addressed the topic of responsible parenthood in an address to a gathering of families in 1994:

> The Church's teaching about "responsible parenthood" is based on this essential anthropological and ethical foundation. Unfortunately, *Catholic thought is often misunderstood* on this point, as if the Church supported an ideology of fertility at all costs, urging married couples to procreate indiscriminately and without thought for the future. But one need only study the pronouncements of the Magisterium to know that this is not so.
>
> Truly, in begetting life the spouses fulfil one of the highest dimensions of their calling: they are *God's co-workers*. Precisely for this reason they must have an extremely responsible attitude. In deciding whether or not to have a child, they must not be motivated by selfishness or carelessness, but by a prudent, conscious generosity that weighs the possibilities and circumstances, and especially gives priority to the welfare of the unborn child. Therefore, when there is a reason not to procreate, this choice is permissible and may even be necessary. However, there remains the duty of carrying it out with criteria and methods that respect the total truth of the marital act in its unitive and procreative dimension, as wisely regulated by nature itself in its biological rhythms. One can comply with them and use them to advantage, but they cannot be "violated" by artificial interference.[355]

---

354 Pope John Paul II, 'Holy Mass at the Capital Mall' Homily, 7 October 1979, n. 6, http://www.vatican.va/holy_father/john_paul_ii/homilies/1979/documents/hf_jp-ii_hom_19791007_usa-washington_en.html (accessed 2010-2014).

355 Pope John Paul II, 'Parents are God's Co-workers', *L'Osservatore Romano*, 20 July 1994.

Appendix A: The Population Question

During the Jubilee of Families in 2000, Pope John Paul II returned to the topic saying:

> To cooperate with God in the transmission of life requires a responsible use of sexuality. For just reasons, spouses may wish to space the births of their children. It is their duty to make certain that their desire is not motivated by selfishness but is in conformity with the generosity appropriate to responsible parenthood. When it is a question of harmonizing married love with the responsible transmission of life, the morality of the behavior does not depend on sincere intention and evaluation of motives alone; but it must be determined by objective criteria, criteria drawn from the nature of the person and his acts, criteria that respect the total meaning of mutual self-giving and human procreation. Periodic continence, that is, the methods of birth regulation based on self-observation and the use of the infertile periods, is in conformity with the objective criteria of morality. In this context the couple comes to experience how conjugal communion is enriched with those values of tenderness and affection which constitute the inner soul of human sexuality, in its physical dimension also.[356]

In an address to the UN Human Rights Council in September 2011, Archbishop Silvano M. Tomasi, Vatican observer to the U.N. in Geneva, said that parents should have the freedom to decide how many children they have without any government involvement. Couples in every country need "the liberty to decide responsibly, free from all social or legal coercion, the number of children they will have and the spacing of their births." He said:

---

[356] Pope John Paul II, 'Children, Springtime Of The Family And Society', Rome, 14-15 October 2000, http://www.vatican.va/roman_curia/pontifical_councils/family/documents/rc_pc_family_doc_20001014_rome-jubilee-of-families-index_en.html#Responsibility in Transmitting Life and Protecting Children (accessed 26 September 2011).

> It should not be the intent of governments or other agencies to decide for couples but, rather, to create the social conditions which will enable them to make appropriate decisions in the light of their responsibilities to God, to themselves, and to the society of which they are part.[357]

The Church gives no direct guidance to couples about how many children they should have. They are entitled to make decisions taking into account the resources needed to care for their children. They may take into account the needs of the community in which they find themselves, their national community, or the world community. In circumstances in which we face an ageing population and a birth rate in a country like Australia that is well below replacement level, there is an argument for having a family size above, or even well above, the replacement level of 2.1 depending on the circumstances of the family. If some families do not increase their family size then the ageing population issue is only going to get worse. We will lack sufficient people in employment to care for, and for their taxes to fund the care of, people who are no longer able to work, including people who are aged and people who have disabilities.

From an international perspective you might argue that large family size is irresponsible because of its contribution to the overall growth rate that may challenge sustainability and the availability of the resources needed to feed, clothe and shelter populations; perhaps making Australia a less welcoming place for people seeking asylum after having been displaced from their own countries. Rather than increasing our own birth rate, perhaps we should be taking in more refugees. However, there is certainly room to move between these two positions, especially with Australia's birth rate being so low.

---

[357] 'Government should not decide family size, Vatican observer insists', *EWTN News*, 17 September 2011, http://www.ewtnnews.com/catholic-news/World.php?id=3982 (accessed 26 September 2011).

Appendix A: The Population Question

Ultimately, family size is a decision that a couple must make in relation to their community or the world community, taking into account their own resources and ability to provide the care that their children may need, the security of their employment and their state of health. I recall having this conversation with Dr John Billings in relation to our own decisions. His advice was that, apart from spacing children so that you could care for them adequately, you will know when it is time to plan your last child. In other words the resource factors will become more evident and determinative.

The Church's concern in the making of these decisions is more about how they may be implemented and the importance of couples having access to fertility awareness methods. There should always be a good reason to abstain during a potentially fertile time. While there are many factors why, at any one time, a couple may decide not to express their love in the marriage act, the decision to avoid fertility is a very serious decision because it is one of the divine purposes for the marriage act.

An important aspect of all of this is the confidence that we can have now in the ability to identify ovulation, peak fertility and periods of infertility during the cycle. Earlier generations, who relied on the so-called "rhythm method", did not have our advantages because many women had irregular cycles or would certainly develop irregular cycles after birth, during times of stress and during the time of peri-menopause. The development of fertility awareness methods that are reliant upon the woman's symptoms, not the calendar, have made a great deal of difference. As a matter of loyalty to the Church it is also important that married couples make clear that this is the case, and not manufacture pressure on priests and theologians by claiming falsely that the signs and symptoms of infertility, ovulation and possible fertility are not easily recognized. The evidence shows very strongly that this is not the case. Given the current state of knowledge, it is simply untrue to claim that there are some couples who are unable to use natural family planning effectively. The pregnancy rates are comparable to the most effective of the contraceptive methods.[358]

There is a great deal of richness for the relationship of a couple who practise fertility awareness or natural family planning. The abstinence required ensures that they develop a real friendship and not just a sexual relationship. The crucial significance of not suppressing fertility is that the couple's love-making can be a genuine witness to God's love. There is a sacramental significance in their love being a witness to God's love, a love that is both unitive and fruitful: a love that is a complete gift of one to the other according to the divine plan of forming one flesh unity and, at the same time, being open to the possibility of new life and of cooperating with God in the coming to be of that new life.

As Christians, we understand that we find fulfilment and express our personalities in the complete gift of ourselves and of love to another. In marriage, there is both *agape* in the giving and *eros* in the desire for the other's love. Both *eros* and *agape* are aspects of divine love as Pope Benedict teaches in his encyclical *Deus Caritas Est*.[359] It is wonderful that in being married we can seek perfection, the perfection of divine love through the marital act. In giving ourselves completely in love and receiving the other completely in love we are giving full expression to the Scriptural understanding of being made in the image and likeness of God, the love of the Persons of the Trinity, and the love of the Persons of the Trinity for us. Marriage has three purposes: the unity of mutual love, the openness to the gift of life and, in the expression of those two purposes, its sacramental meaning and vocation to be a witness to God's love which is both unitive and fruitful.

---

358 Nicholas Tonti-Filippini and Mary Walsh, 'Post-coital Intervention: From Fear of Pregnancy to Rape Crisis', *National Catholic Bioethics Quarterly*, vol. 4, no. 2, 2004.
359 Pope Benedict XVI, *Deus Caritas Est*, op. cit.

Appendix A: The Population Question

As Pope Paul VI expressed it:

> Marriage, then, is far from being the effect of chance or the result of the blind evolution of natural forces. It is in reality the wise and provident institution of God the Creator, whose purpose was to effect in man His loving design. As a consequence, husband and wife, through that mutual gift of themselves, which is specific and exclusive to them alone, develop that union of two persons in which they perfect one another, cooperating with God in the generation and rearing of new lives.[360]

In the light of revelation of the nature of God's love, it is very plain that to suppress fertility in relation to the marriage act would be to render the act less significant as an expression of sacramental meaning: it would cease to be like God's love because it would cease to be fruitful. It would be a rejection of that co-operation with the divine goodness in being open to a new life. So, however a couple resolves the issue of how many children they should have and how they might space them, there is no need to have recourse to methods of family planning that involve suppressing the life-giving capacity of the marriage act or of their bodies or, even worse, adopting methods that suppress life already begun.

---

[360] Pope Paul VI, *Humanae Vitae*, 25 July 1968, n. 8.

Appendix B: Climate Change

1. The Debate in Context

The climate change debates are beset by polemics and politicization so that it is very difficult for a moderately well educated person to know what to believe. Whom can we accept as a reliable authority? How can we assess the competing claims? The purpose of this chapter is to try to elucidate ethical principles that might help guide our responses, whatever decisions we make about the claims made about climate change, the potential consequences of it, possible good effects as well as the bad effects most warned about, and the possible or probable effects of human contribution to it.

Responsible people have long recognized the problems of pollution and the over-use of finite resources such as fossil fuel reserves. Seemingly, in the last decade, awareness of our moral responsibilities in those respects has taken a back seat to the shrill bi-polarity of the climate change debate. Being a climate change sceptic should not mean not being concerned about pollution of land, water and air, or about the need to find sustainable energy sources and to reduce consumption of non-sustainable resources. As Christians, we have particular obligations to respect the created environment and to exercise responsible stewardship. That is the role specified in Scripture, and it reflects our respect for the worth, dignity and wellbeing of our children and grandchildren, and their children and grandchildren. We ought not to weigh down future generations with the burdens of our profligacy.

The climate change debate is but one aspect of our stewardship and should not exclude all others. It is, however, sad that we seem to have lost confidence in the objectivity of the physical sciences.

Appendix B: Climate Change

We have long learned to be sceptical of claims made in the biomedical sciences, fraught as they are by competing financial interests and the possibilities and the realities of influencing human behaviour to embrace, in a large scale way, the new technologies especially in relation to the pharmaceutical industry. One only has to look at the weight loss industry, so successful in selling products and successful, in a sense, because it is unsuccessful. If the technologies sold actually worked, they would have lost their markets! Other examples are the widespread take up of the use of *statins* for the worried well but middle-aged and elderly, and the use of contraceptives despite the availability of fertility awareness methods which are comparably successful in planning family size and spacing, without the side effects.

2. The Intergovernmental Panel on Climate Change (IPCC)
The IPCC assessed the following topics:

- the observed changes in climate and their effects on natural and human systems, regardless of their causes;
- the causes of the observed changes;
- projections of future climate change and related impacts under different scenarios;
- adaptation and mitigation options over the next few decades and their interactions with sustainable development;
- the relationship between adaptation and mitigation on a more conceptual basis with a longer-term perspective;
- the major robust findings and remaining key uncertainties in this assessment.[361]

Obviously the issue is firstly whether there is or is not to be

---

361 IPCC, 'Synthesis Report', *Fourth Assessment Report: Climate Change 2007*, retrieved from https://www.ipcc.ch/publications_and_data/ar4/syr/en/contents.html (accessed 2010-2014).

climate change and, if there is, we need to know what the effects of climate change will be. Secondly, we need to know whether climate change is an inevitable natural process of change. Thirdly, we need to know whether human activities have a significant additional impact on the rate of that change or the severity of the consequences of that change. If human activities do have significant impact on harmful climate change we need to know what aspects of human activities need to change in order to reduce the harm that we might otherwise do. Finally, we need to address the political and economic realities of seeking to bring about change in the factors that influence climate change. There is a moral issue in our taking responsibility for the effects that we have on the future environment and the injustice of leaving to future generations an environment that we have damaged.

An issue that has emerged is who is a reliable source of information on these matters. The IPCC has been criticized. However, their reports would seem to be a good place to start while noting the criticisms and any questions over credibility of the panel and the critics. We do need to reach an opinion on the above matters. The panel reports the following observations:[362]

- Eleven of the last twelve years (1995-2006) rank among the 12 warmest years in the instrumental record of global surface temperature (since 1850). The updated 100-year linear trend (1906 to 2005) of 0.74°C [0.56°C to 0.92°C] is therefore larger than the corresponding trend for 1901 to 2000 given in the TAR [third assessment report] of 0.6°C [0.4°C to 0.8°C]. The linear warming trend over the last 50 years of 0.13°C [0.10°C to 0.16°C] per decade is nearly twice that for the last 100 years. The total temperature increase from 1850-1899

---

362 IPCC, 'Working Group I: The Physical Science Basis', *Fourth Assessment Report: Climate Change 2007*, retrieved from https://www.ipcc.ch/publications_and_data/ar4/wg1/en/spmsspm-direct-observations.html (accessed 2010-2014).

Appendix B: Climate Change

to 2001-2005 is 0.76°C [0.57°C to 0.95°C]. Urban heat island effects are real but local, and have a negligible influence (less than 0.006°C per decade over land and zero over the oceans) on these values.

- New analyses of balloon-borne and satellite measurements of lower- and mid-tropospheric temperature show warming rates that are similar to those of the surface temperature record and are consistent within their respective uncertainties, largely reconciling a discrepancy noted in the TAR.
- The average atmospheric water vapour content has increased since at least the 1980s over land and ocean as well as in the upper troposphere. The increase is broadly consistent with the extra water vapour that warmer air can hold.
- Observations since 1961 show that the average temperature of the global ocean has increased to depths of at least 3000 metres and that the ocean has been absorbing more than 80% of the heat added to the climate system. Such warming causes seawater to expand, contributing to sea level rise.
- Mountain glaciers and snow cover have declined on average in both hemispheres. Widespread decreases in glaciers and ice caps have contributed to sea level rise (ice caps do not include contributions from the Greenland and Antarctic Ice Sheets).
- New data since the TAR now show that losses from the ice sheets of Greenland and Antarctica have very likely contributed to sea level rise over 1993 to 2003. Flow speed has increased for some Greenland and Antarctic outlet glaciers, which drain ice from the interior of the ice sheets. The corresponding increased ice sheet mass loss has often followed thinning, reduction or loss of ice shelves or loss of floating glacier tongues. Such dynamical ice loss is sufficient to explain most of the

Antarctic net mass loss and approximately half of the Greenland net mass loss. The remainder of the ice loss from Greenland has occurred because losses due to melting have exceeded accumulation due to snowfall.

Changes in Temperature, Sea Level and Northern Hemisphere Snow Cover

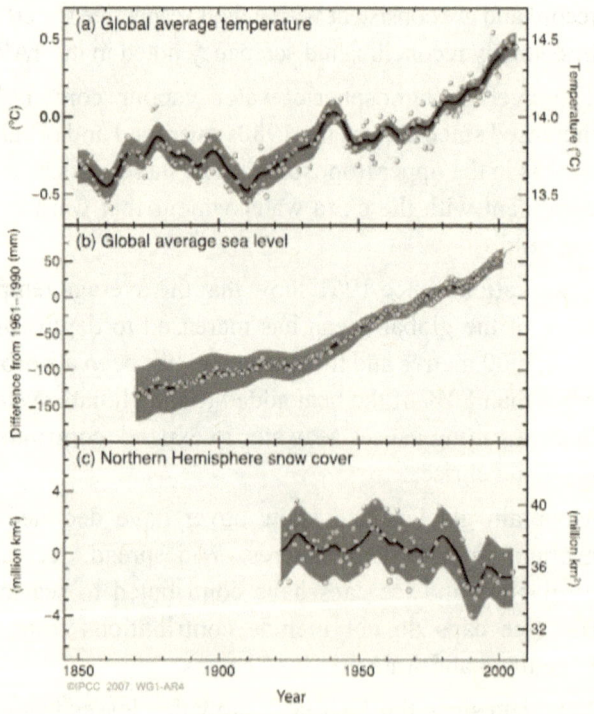

Observed changes in (a) global average surface temperature, (b) global average sea level from tide gauge (blue) and satellite (red) data and (c) Northern Hemisphere snow cover for March-April. All changes are relative to corresponding averages for the period 1961-1990. Smoothed curves represent decadal average values while circles show yearly values. The shaded areas are the uncertainty intervals estimated from a comprehensive analysis of known uncertainties (a and b) and from the time series (c).[363]

---

363 Ibid.

Appendix B: Climate Change

3. Human Contribution to Climate Change

The Australian Parliamentary Library claims that "climate change has often occurred on earth due to natural causes over timescales that vary from decades to hundreds of thousands of years".[364] Nevertheless it reports that:

> ... on the basis of considerable evidence, there is a strong consensus in the climate science research community that the changes that have been observed over the past few decades are mainly caused by human activity. The human influences on climate change arise from combustion of fossil fuels (also known as hydrocarbon fuels) and changes in land use. These activities alter the radiative balance of the earth either by changing its atmospheric composition so as to enhance the natural greenhouse effect, or by changing the reflectivity of the earth's surface or atmosphere.[365]

The main human activities that are claimed to have contributed to an enhancement of the natural greenhouse effect are:[366]

- Combustion of fossil fuels, releasing greenhouse gases.
- Clearing of forests for agriculture, which releases carbon dioxide through increased biomass decay.
- Deforestation, soil tillage and land degradation, which release carbon from the land system and reduce its capacity to absorb and store carbon.

The main human activities that have been claimed to change the reflectivity of the earth's surface and atmosphere are:[367]

---

364 Australian Parliamentary Library, 'Human contribution to climate change', 15 November 2010, http://www.aph.gov.au/About_Parliament/Parliamentary_Departments/Parliamentary_Library/Browse_by_Topic/ClimateChangeold/whyClimate/human/human (accessed 2010-2014).
365 Ibid.
366 Ibid.
367 Ibid.

- Fossil fuel combustion; industrial processes; and biomass burning release aerosols and other pollutants into the atmosphere, changing its capacity to reflect or absorb solar radiation. These aerosols may also be deposited onto the land surface and cause changes to the surface albedo.[368]
- Deforestation, agricultural practices and urbanization change the reflectivity of the earth's surface.

It is also stated:

> Some of these influences can have a cooling effect on the earth's surface and lower atmosphere. For example, most aerosols emitted into the atmosphere reflect solar radiation back out to space. Black carbon particles are an exception, as they strongly absorb heat, and when deposited on snow can act as a significant heat sink on the surface that encourages snow melt. Deforestation tends to increase the albedo of the land surface, since green, hydrated leaves reflect less solar radiation than bare earth. This too contributes a negative or cooling effect to the earth's radiative balance.
>
> There are also complex interactions and feedbacks between many of these processes that are not well understood. For example, while aerosols in the atmosphere contribute a direct cooling effect, they also have an indirect contribution through their effect on the formation and properties of clouds, changing their albedo and lifetime.
>
> However, it is clear that the warming factors are dominant and the net effect of human activities is a warming of the planet. The single most important influence is the increase in greenhouse gas concentrations due to fossil fuel combustion. The figure below illustrates the relative contribution of various processes to radiative forcing of the earth's climate between 1750 and 2005, including the influence of natural changes in solar irradiance.[369]

---

368 Reflective power
369 Ibid.

Appendix B: Climate Change

There are thus human factors that contribute to cooling, such as aerosols in the upper atmosphere, and factors that contribute to heating such as carbon dioxide. The IPCC represented the various human factors between 1750 and 2005 with the following diagram:

Changes in atmospheric constituents and in radiative forcing

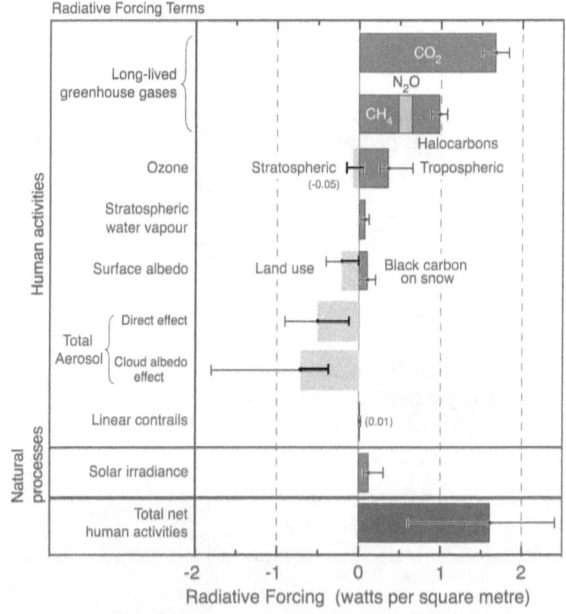

All these radiative forces result from one or more factors that affect climate and are associated with human activities or natural processes. The values represent the forcings in 2005 relative to the start of the industrial era (about 1750). Human activities cause significant changes in long-lived gases, ozone, water vapour, surface albedo (reflective nature), aerosols and contrails (their effect on cloud formation). The only increase in natural forcing of any significance between 1750 and 2005 occurred in solar irradiance. Positive forcings lead to warming of climate and negative forcings lead to a cooling. The thin black line in the diagram attached to each coloured bar represents the range of uncertainty for the respective value.[370]

---

370 IPCC, 'Working Group I: The Physical Science Basis', *Fourth Assessment Report: Climate Change 2007*, chapter 2, figure 2.20, p. 203.

Faith, Science and the Environment

The main sources of the anthropogenic greenhouse gases and their relative contribution to the enhanced greenhouse effect are listed in the table below:[371]

Gas	Principal anthropogenic sources	Lifetime	Proportional contribution to the enhanced greenhouse effect
Carbon dioxide (CO_2)	Fossil fuel burning, biomass burning, gas flaring, cement production, land use and land use change	50–200 years	56 %
Methane (CH_4)	Disturbance of wetlands, rice paddies, ruminant livestock, venting from natural gas wells, biomass burning and decomposition, coal mining, rubbish tips	12 years	16 %
Nitrous oxide (N_2O)	Fossil fuel combustion, fertiliser production, biomass burning	114 years	5 %
Halocarbons (combined)	Industrial production, consumer goods (aerosol can propellants, refrigerants, foam-blowing agents, solvents, fire retardants)	2 to 50,000 years (e.g. CFC-11 is 45 years, CF_4 is 50,000 years)	11 %
Tropospheric ozone (O_3)	Emissions of precursors (carbon monoxide, nitrogen oxides, volatile organic compounds) from fossil fuel combustion and biomass burning	Short-lived	12 %

---

[371] Ibid., table 2.12, p. 204.

Appendix B: Climate Change

The Australian Parliamentary Library concludes:

> The way in which we use the land and change the pattern of vegetation alters the reflectivity of the planet's surface and may reduce or promote the ability of soil and vegetation to absorb, store and release carbon and carbon dioxide.
>
> In agriculture, activities such as land-clearing, burning, deforestation and tillage can change the reflectivity and texture of the land surface, and hence the levels of absorbed radiation, evaporation and evapotranspiration. Changes to soil structure through tillage and removal of vegetation – particularly deforestation – reduce the land's capacity to absorb carbon dioxide. Removal of vegetation also reduces the ability of soils to retain moisture and may make it harder for rainwater to infiltrate, commonly exacerbating erosion. The decay of plant biomass, often associated with processes used in land clearing, contributes to CO_2 and methane emissions.
>
> Changes in soil structure, soil moisture loss and over-cultivation can also reduce soil organic content by reducing the density of soil organisms and accelerating oxidation of organic carbon compounds to produce carbon dioxide. Modified farming practices can help retain soil carbon and hence maximize the potential of soil to act as a carbon sink.
>
> The soil is thought to contain about twice the amount of carbon as the atmosphere. Some proponents of carbon sequestration in soil claim that if regenerative agriculture were practised on the planet's 1.4 billion tillable hectares, it could sequester up to 40 per cent of current CO_2 emissions.[372]

---

372 Australian Parliamentary Library, op. cit.

4. What Needs to Be Done According to the Experts

In 2006, the United Kingdom commissioned an economic analysis by the leading economist, Sir Nicholas Stern:

> [T]he *Review* estimates that if we don't act, the overall costs and risks of climate change will be equivalent to losing at least 5% of global GDP each year, now and forever. If a wider range of risks and impacts is taken into account, the estimates of damage could rise to 20% of GDP or more ... Our actions now and over the coming decades could create risks ... on a scale similar to those associated with the great wars and the economic depression of the first half of the 20th century.[373]

The *Review* supports the creation of a price for carbon, claiming: "Creating a transparent and comparable carbon price signal around the world is an urgent challenge for international collective action." The *Review* argues that it is critical to have a harmonized carbon tax or similar regulatory device both to provide incentives to individual firms and households and to stimulate research and development in low-carbon technologies. Carbon prices must be raised to transmit the social costs of greenhouse gas emissions to the everyday decisions of billions of firms and people.[374]

The Stern Review assumes intergenerational equality. In other words, the cost to be borne by current and future generations should be the same. In the jargon that is used this assumption is referred to as an assumption of zero social discounting. Discounting, in this context, refers to shifting the price to be paid

---

[373] Sir Nicholas Stern, 'Stern Review on the Economics of Climate Change', 2006, retrieved from http://www.hmtreasury.gov.uk/independent_reviews/stern_review_economics_climate_change/sternreview_index.cfm (accessed 5 October 2011).

[374] William D. Nordhaus, 'A Review of the Stern Review on the Economics of Climate Change', *Journal of Economic Literature*, American Economic Association, vol. 45(3), 2007, pp. 686-702, retrieved from http://www.nber.org/papers/w12741 (accessed 2010-2014).

to future generations and is consistent with what is referred to as "ramping up", the idea that adjusting economies in order to reduce carbon can start relatively slowly and gradually increase. This involves making future generations pay proportionately more than current generations. The assumption that Nicholas Stern took is that the cost should be evenly shared and that we should not expect future generations to pay for our profligacy. There is, of course, a philosophical argument to be had over this issue of equality.

Basically, the *Review* is a summary of the case for claiming that there is climate change, that human activities are contributing to it and to the severity of its effects, and that there is a need to change our activities; the latter can be achieved by governments charging a price for carbon use that releases carbon dioxide into the atmosphere. The belief is that the economic pressure will cause changes to what we do, including developing alternative forms of energy rather than burning fossil fuels, so that we produce less carbon dioxide. The moral argument is that we should share the cost of managing to reduce our carbon footprint with future generations rather than impose the cost unfairly on them. Secondly, some of the argument is about urgency – the more we fail to reduce, the greater the burden of climate change on future generations.

5. Criticisms of Climate Change Orthodoxy

The accuracy of IPCC climate projections has been questioned. It is argued by some scientists that it is not possible to project global climate accurately enough to justify the ranges projected for temperature and sea-level rise over the next century. This group of scientists is not necessarily claiming that the IPCC claims are wrong or inflated, just that the evidence depends on modelling and the latter may be inaccurate.

Some scientists reject the IPCC claims about human contribution to climate change. Others have simply said that the causes of global warming are unknown. In other words, the latter accepts the evidence of climate change but not the IPCC claims about human contribution. They claim that it is not possible to determine whether the changes are man-made or natural.

A further group of scientists accepts climate change but believes that it will not all be negative. They blame the IPCC for highlighting only the negative results and argue that, in fact, there could be a net benefit.

There has also been a range of criticisms that are much more specific, targeting what they claim are IPCC errors in reporting and particular uses of data.

The best source of criticism of the IPCC that I could find was from a group called the Non-Government International Panel on Climate Change (NIPCC).[375] They seem to be a large group holding respected positions in relevant scientific fields. They published a report "Climate Change Reconsidered". Their criticisms are not to completely dismiss the IPCC but to raise doubts about the accuracy of modelling and consequentially the conclusions drawn, mostly about human effects on climate change and about whether the effects of climate change will be on-balance negative. One of their general criticisms is about the political nature of the IPCC and its composition, mostly scientists appointed by and thus linked to governments rather than being independent, and its advocating for a view rather than representing the balance or range of scientific opinion.

The first set of concerns NIPCC expresses are about the IPCC modelling for forecasting. They claim that the IPCC violates many of the rules and procedures required for scientific forecasting, making its "projections" of little use to policymakers. Secondly, they question the effect of increasing atmospheric CO_2 on the

---

[375] NIPCC, *Climate Change Reconsidered*, The Heartland Institute, 2009, http://www.nipccreport.org/reports/2009/2009report.html (accessed 2010-2014).

Appendix B: Climate Change

temperature sensitivity of the earth. Thirdly, they review the empirical data on past temperatures. They say that they find no support for the IPCC's claim that climate observations during the 20th century are either unprecedented or provide evidence of an anthropogenic effect on climate. They point to flaws in the famous "hockey-stick" diagram used by the IPCC based on recorded northern hemisphere average temperature changes.[376]

The diagram from the IPCC report includes the following:[377]

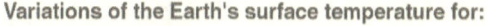
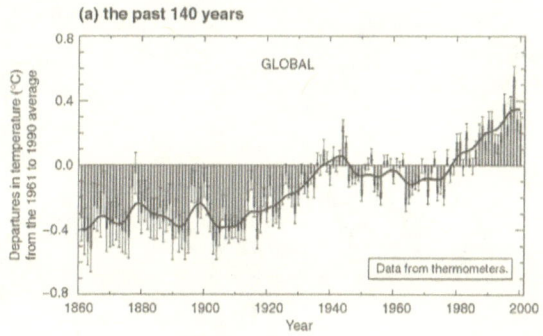
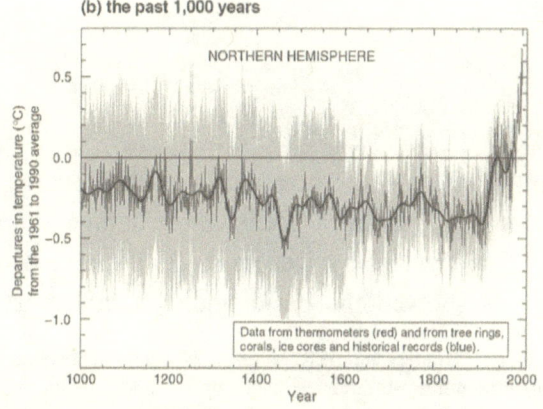

---

376 Ibid., chapter 1.
377 IPCC, 'Working Group I: The Physical Science Basis', *Fourth Assessment Report: Climate Change 2007*, retrieved from http://www.ipcc.ch/ipccreports/tar/wg1/005.htm (accessed 2010-2014).

Critics often refer to the misrepresentation of the medieval period from a single study by Mann et al (1999)[378] and the IPCC's failure to report the authors' uncertainties about the data, based on examining tree ring evidence. The critics claim that there are many studies showing a quite different average temperature for that period. They often refer to the following diagram showing the variations between twelve different studies:[379]

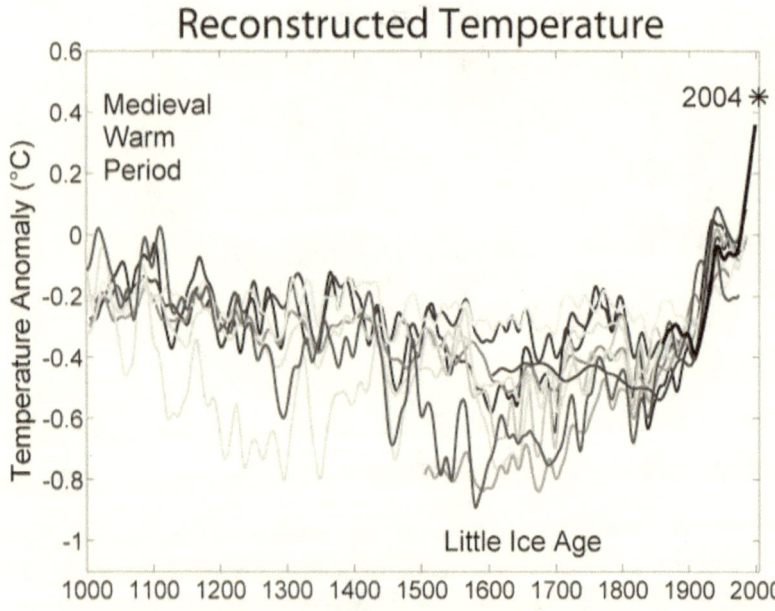

The term "hockey stick graph" has been used for numerous reconstructions of Northern Hemisphere temperatures for the last 600 to 1,000 years: by December 2005 more than a dozen reconstructions showed the basic finding that late 20th century

---

378 M.E. Mann, R.S. Bradley and M.K. Hughes, 'Northern hemisphere temperatures during the past millennium: Inferences, uncertainties, and limitations', *Geophysical Research Letters*, vol. 26, no. 6, 1999, pp. 759-762 (referred to in the IPCC's third report but not in the fourth report).
379 Robert A. Rohde, *1000 Year Temperature Comparison*, 18 November 2005, http://www.globalwarmingart.com/wiki/File:1000_Year_Temperature_Comparison.png (accessed 2010-2014).

Appendix B: Climate Change

temperatures significantly exceeded previous temperatures during that period.

The NIPCC refer to:

> ... the methodological errors of the "hockey stick" diagram of Mann *et al.*, evidence for the existence of a global Medieval Warm Period, flaws in the surface-based temperature record of more modern times, evidence from highly accurate satellite data that there has been no net warming over the past 29 years, and evidence that the distribution of modern warming does not bear the "fingerprint" of an anthropogenic effect.[380]

The NIPCC also challenges the conclusion about the causes of glacier melt. They do not challenge that there is a glacial melt but do say that they could find no evidence of trends that could be attributed to the anthropogenic global warming of the 20th century.[381]

The NIPCC also proposes an alternative theory for climate change. They summarize research of some scientists who say variations in solar activity and sun spots, not greenhouse gases, are the true driver of climate change.[382]

Turning to the issue of the effects of climate change, the NIPCC claim to have debunked IPCC fears that global warming might well cause (or already is causing) more droughts, floods, hurricanes, storms, storm surges, heat waves and wildfires. They point to a lack of support for the IPCC view in the literature.[383]

The NIPCC also discuss the biological effects of rising CO_2 concentrations and warmer temperatures. They claim that these

---

380 NIPCC, op. cit., chapter 3.
381 Ibid., chapter 4.
382 Ibid., chapter 5.
383 Ibid., chapter 6.

effects are unequivocally good news and argue that rising CO_2 levels increase plant growth and make plants more resistant to drought and pests. It is a boon to the world's forests and prairies, as well as to farmers and ranchers and the growing populations of the developing world. These claims seem to me to be more speculative than based on hard evidence.[384]

The NIPCC also discuss the IPCC's claim that CO_2-induced increases in air temperature will cause unprecedented plant and animal extinctions, both on land and in the world's oceans. They say there is little real-world evidence in support of such claims and an abundance of counter evidence that suggests ecosystem biodiversity will *increase* in a warmer and CO_2-enriched world.[385]

Finally, the NIPCC challenge the IPCC's claim that CO_2-induced global warming is harmful to human health. The IPCC blames high-temperature events for increasing the number of cardiovascular-related deaths, enhancing respiratory problems, and fuelling a more rapid and widespread distribution of deadly infectious diseases, such as malaria, dengue and yellow fever. However, the NIPCC claims that a thorough examination of the peer-reviewed scientific literature reveals that further global warming would likely do just the opposite and actually reduce the number of lives lost to extreme thermal conditions. The NIPCC also offer an explanation about how CO_2-induced global warming would help feed a growing global population without major encroachment on natural ecosystems, and how increasing production of biofuels (a strategy recommended by the IPCC) damages the environment and raises the price of food.[386]

As lay persons, all we can do is compare the two sets of claims. Firstly, to see to what extent the critics have disagreed with the

---

384 Ibid., chapter 7.
385 Ibid., chapter 8.
386 Ibid., chapter 9.

Appendix B: Climate Change

IPCC, that is to say how much is left unchallenged of the key propositions that climate change is happening or is likely to be and secondly, that human contribution will make a difference that will increase harm. It becomes a matter of credibility of the competing claims.

Some of the criticism aims to challenge the general credibility of the scholarship of the IPCC by picking up relatively small points; that kind of criticism can be largely put to one side because small errors can usually be found in an academic work, especially one as large as this and which has drawn so much attention. Other criticisms refer to alternative findings that challenge the general propositions, but the question then goes to the credibility of an alternative finding and whether there is a sufficient weight of peer reviewed articles behind it. In science there is hardly a proposition that will not have evidence both for and against it. Much of what happens is the relative weighting of findings by their number and quality of the research.

I am not aiming to draw a conclusion about climate change. I have only tried to summarize the claims made.

BIBLIOGRAPHY

Aquinas, St. Thomas, *Commentary on Aristotle's Physics: Book II*, Lectio 14 (199 a 34-b 33), n. 263, retrieved from http://dhspriory.org/thomas/Physics2.htm#14 (accessed 2010-2014).

Aquinas, St. Thomas, *De Potentiâ*.

Aquinas, St. Thomas, *Questiones Disputatae de Veritate*.

Aquinas, St. Thomas, *Scriptum Super Libros Sententiarum Petri Lombardi*.

Aquinas, St. Thomas, *Summa Contra Gentiles*.

Aquinas, St. Thomas, *Summa Theologiae*.

Aristotle, *Metaphysics*, bk. VII, pt. 7, trans. W.D. Ross, retrieved from http://classics.mit.edu/Aristotle/metaphysics.7.vii.html (accessed 19 November 2011).

Asia for Educators, 'Issues and Trends in China's Demographic History', Columbia University, 2009, http://afe.easia.columbia.edu/special/china_1950_population.htm (accessed 26 September 2011).

Attwood, A., 'Peril in the Square: The Sculpture that Challenged a City', *The Age*, 19 June 2004, http://www.theage.com.au/articles/2004/06/16/1087244973120.html?from=storyrhs (accessed 2010-2014).

Augustine, St., *City of God*.

Augustine, St., *Confessions*.

Augustine, St., *De Trinitate*.

Augustine, St., from his exposition on Psalm 148, retrieved from http://www.goodreads.com/quotes/show/34387 (accessed 10 January 2011).

Augustine, St., *The Catholic and Manichaean Ways of Life*, The Fathers of the Church: A New Translation, vol. 56, trans. D.A. Gallagher and I.J. Gallagher, Boston, Catholic University Press, 1966.

Australian Bureau of Statistics, 'Measures of Australia's Progress', 2009, retrieved from http://betaworks.abs.gov.au/betaworks/betaworks.nsf/projects/MeasuresOfAustralia'sProgress/population/index.htm (accessed 2010-2014).

Australian Catholic Bishops Conference, 'Population in Perspective', Social Justice Statement, 1973.

Bibliography

Australian Government: The Treasury, '2010 Intergenerational Report Overview – Australia's Ageing Population', 2010, http://archive.treasury.gov.au/igr/igr2010/default.asp (accessed 2010-2014).

Australian Institute of Family Studies, 'Fertility and family policy in Australia', Research Paper No. 41, 2008, https://aifs.gov.au/publications/fertility-and-family-policy-australia/2-fertility-rates-demographic-structure-and (accessed 2010-2014).

Australian Parliamentary Library, 'Human contribution to climate change', 15 November 2010, http://www.aph.gov.au/About_Parliament/Parliamentary_Departments/Parliamentary_Library/Browse_by_Topic/ClimateChangeold/whyClimate/human/human (accessed 2010-2014).

Baby Center, 'How many children do you want?' poll, http://www.babycenter.com.au/o4190/how-many-children-do-you-want (accessed 2010-2014).

Baldnerm, S.E. and Carroll, W.E. (trans.), *Aquinas on Creation*, Toronto, Pontifical Institute of Medieval Studies, 1997.

Balthasar, Hans Urs von, *The Glory of the Lord: A Theological Aesthetics, Vol 1 - Seeing the Form*, T&T Clark and Ignatius Press, 1982.

Balthasar, Hans Urs von, *The Glory of the Lord: A Theological Aesthetics, Vol 2 - Studies in Theological Style: Clerical Style*, trans. A. Louth et al, San Francisco, Ignatius Press, 1984.

Barth, K., Bromiley, G.W., and Torrance, T.F., *Church Dogmatics*, vol. 3, pt. 2, New York, T&T Clark, 1960.

BBC News, 'China faces growing gender imbalance', 11 January 2010, http://news.bbc.co.uk/2/hi/8451289.stm (accessed 26 September 2011).

Bente, F. (ed.), *Historical Introductions to the Lutheran Confessions*, retrieved from http://bookofconcord.org/historical-19.php (accessed 3 August 2012).

Bethge, E. (ed.) and Fuller, R.H. (trans.), *Letters and Papers from Prison*, Touchstone, 1997.

Biology Online, 'Genetic Mutations', 2000, http://www.biology-online.org/kb/article.php?p=/2/8_mutations.htm (accessed 2010-2014).

Bourke, V.J. (trans.), *The Essential Augustine*, Indianapolis, Hackett Publishing, 1974.

Bourke, V.J. (trans.), *The Pocket Aquinas*, New York, Washington Square Press, 4th ed., 1965.

Cairns, G., 'Celtic Christianity Homily: The Goodness of Creation', delivered at the Union Community Church in Valparaiso, Indiana, 3 May 2009, http://wn.com/celtic_christianity_homily_the_goodness_of_creation_by_rev_dr_george_cairns (accessed 2010-2014).

Carroll, J., 'Americans: 2.5 Children Is "Ideal" Family Size', 26 June 2007, http://www.gallup.com/poll/27973/americans-25-children-ideal-family-size.aspx (accessed 27 September 2011).

Carson, R., *Silent Spring*, Boston, Houghton Mifflin, 1962.

Catechism of the Catholic Church, St Paul Publications, 2000.

Churton, E. (trans.), *The Early English Church*, London, Burns, 1840.

CIA World Factbook, 'China life expectancy at birth', 2011, retrieved from http://www.indexmundi.com/china/life_expectancy_at_birth.html (accessed 26 September 2011).

Clowney, D., 'Plato's Aesthetics', *Aesthetics*, http://www.rowan.edu/open/philosop/clowney/Aesthetics/philos_artists_onart/plato.htm (accessed 29 December 2010).

Congregation for the Doctrine of the Faith, *Donum Vitae*, English translation: *Instruction on Respect for Human Life in its Origin and on the Dignity of Procreation*, 22 February 1987.

Cooper, A.G., *Naturally Human, Supernaturally God: Deification in Pre-conciliar Catholicism*, US, Fortress Press, 2014.

Council of Vienne 1311-1312 AD, *First Decree*, available at http://www.papalencyclicals.net/Councils/ecum15.htm#can1 (accessed 9 June 2011).

Coyne, Reverend George V., 'Science Does Not Need God. Or Does It?', lecture presented at the American Enterprise Institute, 21 October 2005, http://home.comcast.net/~pdnoerd/DrCoyneTalk.pdf (accessed 2010-2014).

Dante Alighieri, *The Divine Comedy: Paradiso*.

Darwin, Charles, in 1859, *The Origin of the Species by Means of Natural Selection: The descent of man and selection in relation to sex*, repub. by Encyclopaedia Britannica, 1952.

Bibliography

Darwin, Charles, letter to J. Fordyce on 7 May 1879, 'Letter no. 12041', *Darwin Correspondence Project*, http://www.darwinproject.ac.uk/entry-12041 (accessed 2010-2014).

Das Gupta, M. and Bhat, P.N.M., 'Fertility decline and increased manifestation of sex bias in India', *Population Studies*, vol. 51, 1997, pp. 307-315.

Davies, O. (ed.), *Gateway to Paradise / Basil the Great*, trans. T. Witherow, Brooklyn, New City Press, 1991.

Davies, P.C.W and Brown, J.R. (eds.), *The Ghost in the Atom*, Cambridge, Cambridge University Press, 1986.

Dawkins, Richard, *The God Delusion*, Boston, Houghton Mifflin, 2006.

Dawkins, Richard, *The Selfish Gene*, New York, Oxford, 1976.

Dessain, C.S. and Gornall, T. (eds.), *The Letters and Diaries of John Henry Newman*, vol. XXIV, Oxford, Clarendon Press, 1973.

Ding, Q.J., and Hesketh, T., 'Family size, fertility preferences, and sex ratio in China in the era of the one child family policy: results from national family planning and reproductive health survey', *BMJ*, 11 May 2006.

Discovery Institute – Center for Science and Culture, 'What is intelligent design?', *Intelligent Design*, http://www.intelligentdesign.org/whatisid.php (accessed 2010-2014).

Dixon, T., *Science and Religion: A Very Short Introduction*, Oxford University Press, 2008.

Ehrlich, P.R., *The Population Bomb*, N.Y.: Ballantine Books, 1968.

Einstein, A., *Out of My Later Years*, Philosophical Library, New York, 1950.

Elegant, S., 'Why Forced Abortions Persist in China', *Time Magazine*, 30 April 2007.

Evolutionist, 'Beyond Darwin and Neo-Darwinism', *Mechanisms of Evolution*, 31 December 2007, http://mechanismsevo.blogspot.com.au/2007/12/beyond-darwin-and-neo-darwinism.html (accessed 2010-2014).

EWTN News, 'Government should not decide family size, Vatican observer insists', 17 September 2011, http://www.ewtnnews.com/catholic-news/World.php?id=3982 (accessed 26 September 2011).

Ezhilmalai, D., (Union Minister for Health and Family Welfare, Republic of India), statement at The Hague Forum On Review of Progress in the

Implementation of the ICPD Programme-of Action, 9 February 1999, retrieved from http://www.un.org/popin/icpd/icpd5/hague/india.pdf (accessed 26 September 2011).

Feng, G., and Hao, L., 'A summary of family planning regulations for 28 regions in China' [in Chinese], *Population Research*, 4, 1992.

First Vatican Council, *Dogmatic Constitution on the Catholic Faith (Dei Filius) (1869-1870 AD)*.

Francis of Assisi, St., *Little Flowers of St Francis*, trans. R. Brown, New York, Doubleday, 1991.

Frankena, W.K., *Ethics*, 2nd ed., Englewood Cliffs, Prentice Hall 1973, chapter 5, retrieved from http://www.ditext.com/frankena/e5.html (accessed 2010-2014).

Gallagher, D.B., 'The Analogy of Beauty and the Limits of Theological Aesthetics', *Theandros*, vol. 3, no. 3, 2006, retrieved from http://www.theandros.com/beauty.html (accessed 29 December 2010).

Gehring, W.J., 'The genetic control of eye development and its implications for the evolution of the various eye-types', *International Journal of Developmental Biology*, vol. 46, 2002, pp. 65-73.

Gendercide Watch, 'Case Study: Female Infanticide', http://www.gendercide.org/case_infanticide.html (accessed 26 September 2011)

Gould, S.J., *The Structure of Evolutionary Theory*, Cambridge, Belknap Press, 2002.

Granger, I.M., 'The Canticle of Brother Sun', *Poetry Chaikhana*, retrieved from http://www.poetry-chaikhana.com/F/FrancisofAsi/CanticleofBr.htm (accessed 6 August 2011).

Guilmoto, C.Z., 'Characteristics of Sex Ratio Imbalance in India, and Future Scenarios', 4th Asia Pacific Conference on Reproductive and Sexual health and Rights, UNFPA, Hyderabad, India, 29-31 October 2007, http://www.unfpa.org/gender/docs/studies/india.pdf (accessed 26 September 2011).

Halsall, P., 'Fifth Ecumenical Council: Constantinople II, 553', *Medieval Sourcebook*, 1996, http://www.fordham.edu/halsall/basis/const2.html (accessed 29 December 2010).

Hardin, G., 'The Feast of Malthus', *The Social Contract*, Spring 1998, http://www.thesocialcontract.com/cgi-bin/showarticle.pl?articleID=737 (accessed 1 September 2011).

Hawking, Stephen, 'Does God play Dice?', lecture available at http://www.hawking.org.uk/does-god-play-dice.html (accessed 2010-2014).

Hawking, Stephen, *A Brief History of Time*, Bantam Books, 1988.

Heine, R.E. (trans.), *Origen: Homilies on Genesis and Exodus*, Fathers of the Church, vol. 71, Washington, Catholic University of America Press, 1982.

Henig, R.M., *Monk in the Garden: The Lost and Found Genius of Gregor Mendel, the Father of Genetics*, New York, Houghton Mifflin, 2000.

Hesketh, T. and Zhu, W.X., 'The one child family policy: the good, the bad, and the ugly', *BMJ*, 7 June 1997, http://www.ncbi.nlm.nih.gov/pmc/articles/PMC2126838/ (accessed 2010-2014).

Hesketh, T., Lu, L. and Xing, Z.W., 'The effect of China's one-child family policy after 25 years', *New England Journal of Medicine*, 15 September 2005.

Hoffman, B. and Dukas, H. (eds.), *Albert Einstein, the human side*, New Jersey, Princeton, 1979.

Horn, S.O. et al, *Creation and Evolution*, Ignatius Press, 2006.

Horn, S.O., and Wiedenhofer, S., *Creation and Evolution*, trans. M.J. Miller, San Francisco, Ignatius Press, 2007.

Integrated Regional Information Networks (IRIN), 'Philippines: Battle over reproductive health bill intensifies', 17 November 2010, http://www.refworld.org/docid/4ce6834c17.html (accessed 2010-2014).

International Theological Commission, 'Communion and Stewardship: Human Persons Created in the Image of God', *The July 2004 Vatican Statement on Creation and Evolution*, http://www.philvaz.com/apologetics/p80.htm (accessed 2010-2014).

Internet Encyclopedia of Philosophy, 'Origen of Alexandria', http://www.iep.utm.edu/origen-of-alexandria/ (accessed 29 December 2010).

IPCC, *Fourth Assessment Report: Climate Change*, 2007.

Jewish Encyclopedia, 'Philo Judæus', 1906, http://www.jewishencyclopedia.com/view.jsp?artid=281&letter=P#ixzz1LN6CLUdW, (accessed 5 March 2011).

John of Damascus, St., *Writings / Saint John of Damascus*, The Fathers of the Church: A New Translation Vol. 37, trans. F.H. Chase Jr., Washington, Catholic University of America Press, 1970.

Kane, P. and Choi, C.Y., 'China's one child family policy', *BMJ*, 9 October 1999, http://www.ncbi.nlm.nih.gov/pmc/articles/PMC1116810/ (accessed 2010-2014).

Kant, Immanuel, *The Critique of Judgement, Part I: Critique of Aesthetic Judgement*, trans. J.C. Meredith, retrieved from http://ebooks.adelaide.edu.au/k/kant/immanuel/k16j/ (accessed 29 December 2010).

Lam, D., 'Population dynamics and poverty in retrospect', *The World We Want,* 2013, http://www.worldwewant2015.org/node/301885 (accessed 28 July 2014).

Leopold, A., *A Sand County Almanac*, New York, Oxford University Press, 1949.

Lewis, C.S., *The Great Divorce*, 1945.

Liu, T. and Zhang, X., 'Ratio of males to females in China' *BMJ*, 9 April 2009, http://dx.doi.org/10.1136/bmj.b483 (accessed 2010-2014).

Maimonides, M., *The Guide of the Perplexed*, vol. 2, trans. S. Pines, Chicago, University of Chicago, 1963.

Malthus, T.R., *An Essay on the Principle of Population*, New York, Dutton, 1960.

Mann, M.E., Bradley, R.S., and Hughes, M.K., 'Northern hemisphere temperatures during the past millennium: Inferences, uncertainties, and limitations', *Geophysical Research Letters*, Vol. 26, No. 6, 1999.

Mayr, E., *What Evolution Is*, Basic Books, 2001.

McBride, T.M., 'Beauty, Contemplation, and the Virgin Mary', http://www.christendom-awake.org/pages/mcbride/beauty.htm (accessed 5 January 2011).

McBrien, R., 'Sacramentality: A Basic Vision for All', *30 Good Minutes*, program 4214, Chicago Sunday Evening Club, 10 January 1999, retrieved from http://www.csec.org/csec/sermon/McBrien_4214.htm (accessed 2010-2014).

McDonald, D., 'What is the Catholic Position on Creationism and Evolution?', http://www.davidmacd.com/catholic/catholic_creationism.htm, (accessed 2010-2014).

McGrath. A.E. (ed.), *The Christian Theology Reader*, 3rd ed., Blackwell 2007.

Miller, E. (ed.), *Essays: Moral, Political and Literary*, Indianapolis, Liberty, 1985.

Myers, D.N., *Resisting History: Historicism and Its Discontents in German-Jewish Thought*, Princeton, Princeton University Press, 2011.

National Bureau of Statistics of China, 'China's population by age and sex in 1990 (based on 1990 population census)', 1992, retrieved from http://www.china-profile.com/data/fig_p_19a_m.htm (accessed 2010-2014).

National Health and Medical Research Council, *Ethical Guidelines for the Care of People in Unresponsiveness (Vegetative State) or a Minimally Responsive State*, Australian Government, 2008.

National Institute of Child Health & Human Development, 'Down syndrome rates', retrieved from http://web.archive.org/web/20060901004316/http://www.nichd.nih.gov/publications/pubs/downsyndrome/down.htm#Questions, (accessed 9 June 2011).

NationMaster, 'Countries Compared by People > Population growth rate', CIA World Factbooks 2003-2013, http://www.nationmaster.com/graph/peo_pop_gro_rat-people-population-growth-rate (accessed 2010-2014).

New World Encyclopedia, 'Origen', http://www.newworldencyclopedia.org/entry/Origen#Impact (accessed 29 December 2010).

Newman, John Henry, *An Essay on the Development of Catholic Doctrine*, Longman Green & Co., 1878, retrieved from http://www.newmanreader.org/works/development/index.html (accessed 2010-2014).

Newman, John Henry, *The Philosophical Notebook of John Henry Newman*, vol. II, eds. E. Sillem and A. J. Boekrad, Louvain, 1970.

NIPCC, *Climate Change Reconsidered*, The Heartland Institute, 2009, http://www.nipccreport.org/reports/2009/2009report.html (accessed 2010-2014).

Nordhaus, W.D., 'A Review of the Stern Review on the Economics of Climate Change', *Journal of Economic Literature*, American Economic Association, vol. 45(3), 2007, pp. 686-702, retrieved from http://www.nber.org/papers/w12741 (accessed 2010-2014).

O'Neill, D., 'Pre-Darwinian Theories', *Early Theories of Evolution*, http://anthro.palomar.edu/evolve/evolve_1.htm, (accessed 5 March 2011).

Osborn, E.F., *Irenaeus of Lyons*, Cambridge and New York, Cambridge University Press, 2001.

Pagan Aguiar, P.A. and Auer, T. (eds.), *The Human Person and a Culture of Freedom*, Washington, Catholic University Press, 2009.

Pagewise Inc., 'The Cosmological Argument of Aquinas', http://www.essortment.com/all/aquinascosmolog_rend.htm (accessed 2010-2014).

Park, C.B., and Cho, N.H., 'Consequences of son preference in a low fertility society: imbalance of the sex ratio at birth in Korea', *Population and Development Review*, Vol. 21, No. 1, March 1995.

Philippine Senate and House of Representatives, 'RH Bill – Philippines: full text of reproductive health and related measures', May 2010, http://www.likhaan.org/content/rh-bill-philippines-full-text-reproductive-health-and-related-measures (accessed 2010-2014).

Pieper, J., *Faith, Hope, Love*, Chicago, Ignatius Press, 1992.

Plato, *Meno*, trans. B. Jowett, retrieved from http://www.fullbooks.com/Meno.html (accessed 2010-2014).

Plato, *Phaedo*, trans. B. Jowett, retrieved from http://classics.mit.edu/Plato/phaedo.html (accessed 2010-2014).

Plato, *The Republic*, ed. G.R.F. Ferrari, trans. T. Griffith, Cambridge, Cambridge University Press, 2000.

Pontifical Academy for Life, 'Prospects for Xenotransplantation: Scientific Aspects and Ethical Consideration', *L'Osservatore Romano*, 26 September 2001.

Ponting, C., *The Guardian Outlook*, 20 June 1992.

Pope Benedict XVI, *Caritas in Veritate*, 29 June 2009.

Pope Benedict XVI, *Deus Caritas Est*, 25 December 2005.

Pope Benedict XVI, *Fighting Poverty To Build Peace*, 1 January 2009.

Pope Benedict XVI, General Audience, 9 Nov 2005.

Pope Benedict XVI, *If You Want to Cultivate Peace, Protect Creation*, 1 January 2010.

Pope Benedict XVI, *Meeting of the Holy Father Benedict XVI with the Clergy of the Dioceses of Belluno-Feltre and Treviso*, 24 July 2007.

Pope John Paul II, 'Children, Springtime Of The Family And Society', Rome, 14-15 October 2000.

Bibliography

Pope John Paul II, 'General Audience', *L'Osservatore Romano*, 26 January 2000.

Pope John Paul II, 'Holy Mass at the Capital Mall' Homily, 7 October 1979.

Pope John Paul II, 'Parents are God's Co-workers', *L'Osservatore Romano*, 20 July 1994.

Pope John Paul II, 'Theology of the Body' Catechesis, *L'Osservatore Romano*, 31 Mar 1980.

Pope John Paul II, *Centesimus Annus*, 1 May 1991.

Pope John Paul II, *Message for the World Day of Peace, Peace with God the Creator, Peace with All Creation*, 1990.

Pope John Paul II, *Sollicitudo Rei Socialis*, 30 December 1987.

Pope John Paul II, *Truth Cannot Contradict Truth*, 22 October 1996.

Pope John Paul II, *Veritatis Splendor*, 6 August 1993.

Pope Paul VI, *Humanae Vitae*, 25 July 1968.

Pope Paul VI, *Octogesima Adveniens*, 14 May 1971.

Pope Pius XII, *Humani Generis*, 12 August 1950.

Ratzinger, Joseph Cardinal, *'In the beginning ...' A Catholic Understanding of the Story of Creation and the Fall*, Eerdmans, 1995.

Ratzinger, Joseph Cardinal, *The Feeling of Things, the Contemplation of Beauty*, 2002.

Richards, J.R., *Human Nature After Darwin: A Philosophical Introduction*, London, Routledge, 2000.

Right Diagnosis, 'Statistics about Edwards Syndrome', http://www.rightdiagnosis.com/e/edwards_syndrome/stats.htm#medical_stats, (accessed 9 June 2011).

Roberts, A., Donaldson, J. and Coxe, A.C. (eds.), *Ante-Nicene Fathers*, vol. 5, Buffalo, Christian Literature Co., 1886.

Rohde, R.A., '1000 Year Temperature Comparison', 18 November 2005, http://www.globalwarmingart.com/wiki/File:1000_Year_Temperature_Comparison.png (accessed 2010-2014).

Rosenberg, M., 'China's One Child Policy', *About Education*, http://geography.about.com/od/populationgeography/a/onechild.htm (accessed 26 September 2011).

Rosenberg, M., 'India's Population: India Likely to Surpass China In Population by 2030', *About Education*, http://geography.about.com/od/obtainpopulationdata/a/indiapopulation.htm (accessed 26 September 2011).

Santamaria, J.N. and Tonti-Filippini, N. (eds.), *Proceedings of the 1983 Annual Conference of St Vincent's Bioethics Centre*, Melbourne, 1983.

Saward, J., *The Beauty of Holiness and the Holiness of Beauty*, San Francisco, Ignatius Press, 1997.

Schaefer, J., *Theological Foundations for Environmental Ethics*, Georgetown University Press, 2009.

Schaff, P., *History of the Christian Church, Volume II: Ante-Nicene Christianity. A.D. 100-325*, retrieved from http://www.ccel.org/ccel/schaff/hcc2.txt (accessed 29 December 2010).

Schilpp, P. A., (ed.), *The Philosophy of G. E. Moore*, Evanston, Northwestern University Press, 1942.

Schönborn, Christoph Cardinal, 'Finding Design in Nature', *New York Times*, 7 Jul 2005, http://www.millerandlevine.com/km/evol/catholic/schonborn-NYTimes.html (accessed 2010-2014).

Schönborn, Christoph Cardinal, *Chance or Purpose? Creation, Evolution, and a Rational Faith*, San Francisco, Ignatius Press, 2007.

Schure, T., 'China's Gender Imbalance', *Worldpress*, 6 January 2011, http://www.worldpress.org/Asia/3676.cfm#down (accessed 26 September 2011).

Scouteris, C., 'Platonic Elements in Pseudo-Dionysius Anti-Manichaean Ontology', http://www.orthodoxresearchinstitute.org/articles/dogmatics/scouteris_ontology.htm (accessed 2 January 2011).

Second Vatican Council, *Dei Verbum*.

Second Vatican Council, *Gaudium et Spes*.

Second Vatican Council, *Lumen Gentium*.

Shah, A., 'Why Is Biodiversity Important? Who Cares?', *Global Issues*, 2009, http://www.globalissues.org/article/170/why-is-biodiversity-important-who-cares (accessed 2 Dec 2010).

Singer, Peter (ed.), *Applied Ethics*, New York, Oxford University Press, 1988.

Singer, Peter (ed.), *In Defense of Animals: The Second Wave*, Oxford, Blackwell, 2005.

Singer, Peter, *Animal Liberation: Towards an End to Man's Inhumanity to Animals*, Paladin Books, 1977.

Singer, Peter, *Practical Ethics*, 2nd, Cambridge, Cambridge University Press, 1993.

Sorrell, R.D., *St Francis of Assisi and Nature: Tradition and Innovation in Western Christian Attitudes Towards the Environment*, Oxford, Oxford University Press, 1988.

Stanford Encyclopaedia of Philosophy, 'Aesthetic Judgement', 2003, http://plato.stanford.edu/entries/aesthetic-judgment/#1 (accessed 29 December 2010).

Stanford Encyclopaedia of Philosophy, 'Intrinsic vs. Extrinsic Value', 2010, http://plato.stanford.edu/archives/win2010/entries/value-intrinsic-extrinsic, (accessed 2010-2014).

Stanford Encyclopaedia of Philosophy, 'Teleological Notions in Biology', 2003, http://plato.stanford.edu/entries/teleology-biology/#ment (accessed 27 July 2011).

Stephens, W.R.W. (trans.), *Nicene and Post-Nicene Fathers*, First Series, Vol. 9, ed. P. Schaff, Buffalo, Christian Literature Publishing, 1889, retrieved from http://www.newadvent.org/fathers/190112.htm (accessed 2010-2014).

Stern, N., 'Stern Review on the Economics of Climate Change', 2006, retrieved from http://www.hmtreasury.gov.uk/independent_reviews/stern_review_economics_climate_change/sternreview_index.cfm (accessed 5 October 2011).

Taylor, J.H. (trans.), *Ancient Christian Writers 41-42*, New York, Newman Press, 1982.

Taylor, P.W., *Respect for Nature: A Theory of Environmental Ethics*, Princeton University Press, 1986.

Teilhard de Chardin, P., *Christianity and Evolution*, trans. R. Hague, New York, Harcourt, 1971.

The Australian, 'Pope arrives in Spain saying economy not just for profit', 18 August 2011, http://www.theaustralian.com.au/news/world/

pope-arrives-in-spain-saying-economy-not-just-for-profit/story-e6frg6so-1226117727570 (accessed 22 September 2011).

The Canons of the Fourth Lateran Council, 1215, retrieved from http://www.fordham.edu/halsall/basis/lateran4.html (accessed 18 July 2011).

The World Factbook, 'Country Comparison – Total Fertility Rate', Central Intelligence Agency, Washington, 2009, https://www.cia.gov/library/publications/the-world-factbook/rankorder/2127rank.html (accessed 2010-2014).

Theissen, G.E. (ed.), *Theological Aesthetics*, Grand Rapids, Eerdmans, 2006.

Tonti-Filippini, Nicholas and Walsh, Mary, 'Post-coital Intervention: From Fear of Pregnancy to Rape Crisis', *National Catholic Bioethics Quarterly*, vol. 4, no. 2, 2004.

Tonti-Filippini, Nicholas, *About Bioethics Volume III: Transplantation, Biobanks and the Human Body*, Ballan, Connor Court, 2012.

Tonti-Filippini, Nicholas, *About Bioethics Volume IV: Motherhood, Embodied Love and Technology*, Ballan, Connor Court, 2013.

UN Department of Economic and Social Affairs, 'What would it take to accelerate fertility decline in the least developed countries?', *UN Population Division Policy Brief*, March 2009, http://www.un.org/esa/population/publications/UNPD_policybriefs/UNPD_policy_brief1.pdf (accessed 1 September 2011).

UN Department of Economic and Social Affairs, Population Division (2007), 'Table A.8 – average annual rate of population change by country', *World Population Prospects: The 2006 Revision*, retrieved from http://www.un.org/esa/population/publications/wpp2006/WPP2006_Highlights_rev.pdf (accessed 2010-2014).

UN Economic and Social Council, 'World population monitoring, focusing on the contribution of the Programme of Action of the International Conference on Population and Development to the internationally agreed development goals, including the Millennium Development Goals – Report of the Secretary-General', Commission on Population and Development: Forty-second session, item 3 of the provisional agenda, 2009, [E/CN.9/2009/3], https://documents-dds-ny.un.org/doc/UNDOC/GEN/N09/212/29/PDF/N0921229.pdf?OpenElement (accessed 2010-2014).

Bibliography

UN Population Division, 'Guidelines on Reproductive Health', Population Information Network (POPIN), http://www.un.org/popin/unfpa/taskforce/guide/iatfreph.gdl.html (accessed 2010-2014).

United Nations Family Planning Association (UNFPA), Programme of Action of the International Conference on Population and Development, Cairo, 1994, summary retrieved from http://ngosbeyond2014.org/articles/2011/10/1/summary-of-the-programme-of-action.html (accessed 2010-2014).

United Nations Family Planning Association (UNFPA), *State of World Population report: People and Possibilities in a World of 7 Billion*, 2011, retrieved from http://www.unfpa.org/publications/state-world-population-2011 (accessed 2010-2014).

University of Michigan, 'The Process of Speciation, Introduction to Global Change', 2002, http://www.globalchange.umich.edu/globalchange1/current/lectures/speciation/speciation.html (accessed 2010-2014).

Wade, M., 'Youthful India may reap age dividend', *The Age*, 27 September 2011, retrieved from http://www.theage.com.au/business/youthful-india-may-reap-age-dividend-20110926-1kto9.html#ixzz1Z7oJTMpI (accessed 2010-2014).

Wang, J.Y., 'Evaluation of the fertility of Chinese women during 1990-2000', *Theses collection of 2001 national family planning and reproductive health survey*, Beijing, China Population Publishing House, 2003.

White, L., 'The Historical Roots of Our Ecological Crisis', http://www.zbi.ee/~kalevi/lwhite.htm (accessed 2010-2014).

Wigner, E., 'The Unreasonable Effectiveness of Mathematics in the Natural Sciences', in *Communications in Pure and Applied Mathematics*, vol. 13, No. I (February 1960), New York, John Wiley & Sons, 1960.

Wilson, E.O., *Sociobiology: The New Synthesis*, Cambridge, Mass., Harvard University Press, 1975.

Winther, R.G., 'Systemic Darwinism', *Proceedings of the National Academy of Sciences U.S.A.*, vol. 105 no. 33, 2008.

World Bank statistics, 'Fertility rate, total (births per woman)', 2011, http://data.worldbank.org/indicator/SP.DYN.TFRT.IN?cid=GPD_11 (accessed 26 September 2011).

INDEX[1]

a priori judgments, 149
abortion, 65, 108, 119, 226-227, 232, 241, 243-244, 246, 248, 251, 253, 256-258
Adam and Eve, 95-96, 118, 124
adaptation, 24, 39, 53, 58, 271
aesthetics, 151, 154
agape, 130, 132-133, 268
anamnesis, 149-150
animals, 6-7, 24, 26-28, 34, 38, 47, 64, 67, 77, 94-97, 114, 117, 124-128, 132, 139, 177, 180-181, 187, 189-192, 203-209, 212-213, 217-219
anthropocentrism, 6, 106, 117, 121, 134, 137, 139
Aristotle, 82-83, 110, 150, 247
art
  music, 152, 162, 168-170, 174
  painting, 99, 168, 174
  sculpture, 174
  work of, 152, 155, 157, 168-170
asexual reproduction, 26
atheism, 21
atmosphere, 3-4, 114, 134, 152, 275-279, 281
Averroes, 77
Avicenna, 86-86

baby boomers, 238
Barth, Karl, 44, 60
Beauty, 100, 147, 153, 155, 158, 162-167, 169-170

Being
  eternal, 84
  temporal, 60, 84, 88
Big Bang Theory, 27, 29, 56, 90, 186
Billings, Dr John, 267
biocentrism, 138
biodiversity, 5, 24, 136, 138, 286
biological
  diversity, 14
  species concept, 52
birth rates, 7, 223, 225, 234-235, 238, 241, 259-261
Boethius, 38, 201, 206
Bonhoeffer, Dietrich, 15
Breuer, Isaac, 40
Brunner, Emil, 154

Cairns, Rev Dr George, 141
carbon
  dioxide, 4, 275, 277, 279, 281
  emissions, 3-4
  trading, 4
Caritas in Veritate, 103, 144, 245, 248
Carson, Rachel, 4
Catechism of the Catholic Church, 45, 79, 91
Catholic Church, 9, 12, 14, 118, 189, 243-244, 246
China
  one child policy, 250, 252, 254-255

---

1 Bibliography and footnotes are not included in this index, nor are words such as creation, faith, death, human being and love which occur frequently throughout the text.

chivalry, 212, 214
chromosomes, 25-26
climate change, 1-4, 114, 136, 147, 186, 225, 270-272, 275, 280-282, 285, 287
Cohen, Hermann, 40
conception, 2, 43, 46, 65, 91, 97, 160, 183
consciousness, 23, 43, 59, 70, 99, 105, 141, 149, 203, 209
consequentialism, 117
contemporary physics, 22-23
contraception, 226-227, 232, 241-242, 244, 246, 248, 254-255, 258
Cooper, Adam, 221
cosmological argument, 109
cosmos, 20, 22-23, 90, 109, 145, 172-173, 193, 219
Council of Vienne, 43-44, 60-61, 68, 91-92, 160
Coyne, Dr George, 18-20, 26, 29
creationism, 46, 189
Credo of the People of God, 92
cynicism, 8

Darwin, Charles, xiii, 1, 12, 15-18, 20, 23-24, 28-29, 31, 34, 37-38, 46-51, 53, 55, 57, 111, 114, 186, 188
Dawkins, Richard, xiii, 40-42, 57, 186
de Lamarck, Jean-Baptiste Chevalier, 38-39
deforestation, 134, 136, 279
deification, 174-175, 209, 221-222
deism, 35
Deus Caritas Est, 127, 143, 268

Dionysius, 154, 162-164
divine
  causality, 30, 32, 78
  law, 116, 119
divinity, 162, 182
DNA, 11, 14, 26, 51
dominion, 6, 102, 105, 112, 124, 133, 137, 170, 177
Downs Syndrome, 51, 54
Drummond, Henry, 15
dualism, 134, 160

Early Fathers, xii, 1, 5, 40, 69, 148, 158, 177, 184-185
ecology, 106, 114-115, 125, 139, 173, 184-185, 208
economic aid, 231
economic(s), 7, 34, 137, 219, 224-226, 231-234, 237, 244-245, 247-249, 255-256, 259, 262, 272, 280-281
ecosystems, 137, 139, 286
education of
  children, 228
  women, 228, 256
Ehrlich, Paul, 231
Einstein, Albert, 21, 31
emanationism, 35, 85
energy, 3-4, 113-114, 134, 225, 270, 281
environment, 1, 3-8, 20, 24-25, 38-39, 47, 51, 53, 58, 80, 86, 101, 103, 105-106, 111, 113, 116-117, 119, 122, 123-125, 133, 135-137, 140-141, 144-145, 147, 154, 170-174, 184-185, 198, 225, 235, 256, 270, 272, 286

Index

epigenetic change, 25, 39, 53-54
Erb, Heather, 129
Erbrich, Fr Paul, 58
eros, 129-133, 211, 268
eugenics, 71, 228
Eukaryotes, 26
evil, 41, 77, 83, 89, 92-93, 97-98, 118-121, 138, 142, 167, 179, 193, 231
evolution, 1-2, 6, 9-14, 16, 41-42, 46-48, 50-52, 54-55, 57-59, 61-63, 66, 69-72, 80-82, 86-87, 90-91, 93, 97, 106-107, 109, 113, 116, 120, 181, 186-189, 191, 198, 200, 208, 211, 269
evolutionary, 5, 20, 22, 31, 33, 56, 64, 72, 113, 138, 187, 208-209
  biology, 58, 60
  determinism, 103, 144
  theory, 15, 20, 23, 26, 33-34, 50, 52, 56-58, 65, 90-91, 106, 186, 211

Fall (the), 2, 40, 91-93, 95, 97, 104, 118, 120, 190, 192-193
family, 101, 122, 201, 207, 226-227, 248-249, 254-255, 259, 261-263, 266-267
family planning, 8, 225-226, 232-233, 241-244, 248, 251-2, 258, 268-269, 271
  natural, 268
  responsible, 227, 261, 266
fertility, 24, 223, 233, 236, 240-242, 251, 259, 264, 269
  awareness methods, 267-268, 271

rates, 225-226, 234-235, 239-240, 243, 254-256, 260
  regulation of, 241
First Cause, 109-110
First Vatican Council, 61
Fisher, Dr Frank, viii
fossil fuels, 3, 134, 225, 275, 281
Frankena, William, 99-100
Franklin Dam, viii
Franklin River, viii-ix
free will, 2, 67, 87, 180, 187
fundamentalists, 33, 40, 47, 142, 186-187

Galileo, 9
Gallagher, Daniel, 154
Gaudium et Spes, 65-66, 81, 93, 101, 119
gender, 201, 240, 257, 259
  ideology, 256
  imbalance, 7, 254, 259
  ratio, 257
  specific impacts, 253
Genesis, 2, 9, 12-13, 19, 33-34, 37, 40, 64, 74-75, 89, 92, 94, 97, 102, 105-106, 124, 133, 137, 140-141, 182-184, 187-188, 192-194, 200
genetic, 5, 24-26, 31, 39, 42, 48-49, 51-54, 56, 71, 86, 125, 202, 208, 210-211
  mutation, 24
  variation, 31, 51
genetics, 48, 50-51, 208
glacial melt, 285
global warming, 3, 185, 282, 285-286
Gnosticism, 35, 77, 159

"God of the gaps", 15, 32
good, 83, 89, 92, 97, 99-100, 118-119, 125-126, 129, 139-140, 142, 166, 179-180, 193
  instrumental, 99-100
  intrinsic, 99-100, 106, 118, 121, 123, 126, 138, 150,
  moral judgment, 202
Goodness, 123, 127, 140, 162-163, 167
Gordon River, viii-ix
grace, 95, 132, 174, 178, 209, 220, 222
greenhouse, 4
  effect, 134, 275, 278, 280
  gas emissions, 275-276, 278, 285
"greening of India", 247

Hawking, Stephen, 21-22, 40, 186
health, 99, 134, 188, 223, 235, 237, 243-244, 251, 259, 261
  of children, 228, 251
  of women, 228, 241-243
  reproductive, 226, 232, 240-241, 244, 248
Hellenism, 1
heresy, 77, 83, 89, 100
Hitchens, Christopher, xiii, 186
HIV/Aids, 184, 227, 240, 246
hockey stick graph, 284
Holy Spirit, 73, 92, 160
human, 2-4
  dignity, 120, 188, 195, 203
  genome, 5, 42-43, 61, 67, 69, 87, 91, 189, 207
  origin, 2, 9, 11-13, 17, 20, 62-67, 208-209
  person, 2, 5, 13, 32, 43, 64-66, 105, 108, 119-120, 122, 142-143, 151, 167, 172, 188, 193
  rights, 123, 125, 280
Humani Generis, 11, 58, 62, 68, 92
Hume, David, 151, 153, 157-158

imagination, 181
imago Dei, 57, 61, 64, 91, 118, 149, 172, 179, 182, 200, 204, 206
immigration, 230, 234
Incarnation, 10, 72, 142, 162, 175, 191, 206
India, 224, 231, 247, 249-250, 253, 256-261
infanticide, 71
  female, 253, 256-257
intelligent design, 14, 22, 33
intergenerational equality, 280
Intergovernmental Panel on Climate Change (IPCC), 3, 271-272, 277, 281-287,
International Theological Commission, 29, 31, 172
Internet, 70

Jesus Christ, 45, 104, 130, 195
John Paul II Institute, x-xi
judgment, 63, 99, 148-149, 153, 156-158, 202

Kant, Immanuel, 147, 149-151, 153, 155-157
kenosis, 209, 220
kinship, 138, 140, 197, 208, 211

Index

Küng, Hans, 154

Larmarckian evolution, 58
Leopold, Aldo, 138, 140
life expectancy, 249-250, 259-261
Linneaus's original classification, 52
Lombardi, Peter, 82, 85
longevity, 223, 225, 234-237, 242-243, 260

macroevolution, 51
Magisterium of the Church, 65, 108, 264
Maimonides, 77-78
Malthus, Reverend Thomas, 5, 226, 228, 230-231, 248
man, 2, 12, 31, 40, 44, 65-68, 77, 91-93, 96-97, 101-102, 109, 118-119, 126, 130-131, 133-136, 142, 144, 177, 180-183, 187, 189, 192, 194-195, 217-218, 230, 269
Manichaean heresy, 77, 83, 89
marriage, 18, 32, 122, 131, 181-183, 251, 267-269
materialism, 23, 262
McBride, Sr. Thomas Mary, 164-167
meiosis, 25, 50
Mendel, Gregor Johann, 48-50, 86
microbiology, 208
microevolution, 52
Millennium Goals, 240
mining, 114, 151, 278
mitosis, 50
monism, 35

monosomy disorders, 25, 49
Moore, G.E., 100
Morphological species concept, 52
Munro, Professor Hector, xi
"museum argument", 5
mysticism, 213-214

nations
  developed, 4, 239, 247
  developing, 239
  least developed, 240
natural
  law, 14, 27, 29, 109, 186
  order, 22, 30, 120
  selection, 2, 14, 24, 26, 28, 31, 39, 41, 47, 50-51, 53, 55-58, 60, 86, 90-91, 106, 109, 111, 115-116, 185-186, 190, 210
nature, 2, 14-16, 22, 27, 33, 35, 41, 47, 56, 59, 76-77, 80, 87, 103-104, 113, 116, 118, 122, 125, 133-136, 138, 140, 144, 179, 184, 190, 193, 211, 214, 264-265, 269
neo-Darwinian theories, 28-29, 31
New Testament, 40, 130, 183
Newman, Cardinal John Henry, 15-18, 23, 32, 187
Non-Government International Panel on Climate Change (NIPCC), 282, 285-286
non-sustainable fuel, 3, 225, 270
noosphere, 70

Occam's razor, 41
Old Testament, 39-40, 126
Origen of Alexandria, 154, 159-162

overconsumption, 227

pantheism, 35
Peierls, Sir Rudolf, 23
Persons of the Trinity, 268
Philo Judæus, 40
Plato, 147, 149-150, 158-159, 161-162, 247
pleasure, 99, 103, 116-117, 126, 147-148, 153, 155-156, 158, 205, 249
pollution, 3-4, 135-6, 147, 225, 233, 270
Pope Benedict XVI, 12-13, 21, 27, 73-74, 81, 91, 103-104, 122, 127, 129-130, 132-134, 136-137, 143-145, 152, 173, 181, 186, 188, 244, 246, 248, 268
Pope John Paul II, 6, 11, 32, 65, 67, 81, 97, 101-102, 105, 118-119, 124-125, 133-135, 142-143, 172, 182-183, 186-188, 219, 225, 263-265
Pope Paul V, 35
Pope Paul VI, 92, 134-135, 269
Pope Pius XII, 11, 62, 65
population
   ageing of, 226-227, 236-240, 248, 259-261, 266
   control, 228, 232, 244, 248, 253, 256
   growth, 1, 7-8, 224-229, 232, 234-235, 242-251, 254-255, 261, 286
   overpopulation, 5, 226
   policy, 226, 240, 248-249, 253-254, 259
   question, 226-228, 261

rates, 225, 227, 233-237, 239, 243-244, 247, 250-251, 255-256, 259-261, 266
stabilization, 232
post-modernism, 150-151
poverty, 7, 136, 224, 227-228, 232-235, 240, 244, 246-247
prenatal sex determination, 71, 257-258
productivity, 136, 224, 227, 247-248
prokaryotes, 26
protists, 26
puritanism, 153

random variation, 28
rationality, 10, 57, 61, 67, 113, 180, 203
Ratzinger, Cardinal Josef, 73, 152
Ray, John, 38
redemption, 195, 204
relativism, 157
responsible parenthood, 244, 264-265
resurrection of the body, 44-45, 95
Revelation, 65, 69, 93, 142, 145
RNA, 26
Rosenzweig, Franz, 40

sacramentality
   of all creation, 1, 5-6, 176, 179, 193
sacraments, 176, 193, 196
Saward, John, 164
scepticism, 8
Schaefer, James, 185, 208
Schönborn, Cardinal Christoph, 28-29
Schuster, Professor Peter, 27

science, 1, 3-4, 6-13, 15, 19, 27-29, 31-33, 39-43, 46, 48, 57, 62, 65, 67, 69, 73-74, 80-81, 87, 90, 97, 106-108, 110, 112, 139, 172, 174, 184-187, 248, 270-271, 275, 287
Second Vatican Council, 65, 73, 91, 95, 119, 176, 195
Second World War, 238, 247
sentience, 6, 137, 203
sexual reproduction, 26, 43, 49, 56
sexuality, 122, 244, 249, 265
Shah, Anup, 140
Silent Spring, 4
sin, 2, 40, 59, 81, 91, 93-95, 98, 102, 118-121, 124, 131, 146, 162, 175, 179-180, 191, 193, 218, 220, 222
Singer, Peter, 7, 117, 137, 139-140, 198-205
sociobiology, 210-211
Socrates, 149
solar panels, xii-xiii
solidarity, 66, 245
soul
  animal, 91
  evolution of, 58-59, 61, 63, 67, 69
  human, 32, 37-38, 40-43, 60-62, 64-65, 67, 69, 77, 91, 107, 131-132, 181, 186-189
  immortal, 1, 33, 43, 57, 60-61, 64, 81, 91-92, 107, 127, 187, 207
speciation, 24, 52
species, 2, 4-6, 9, 14-16, 18, 20, 24, 27-28, 31-32, 35, 37-38, 43, 46-48, 52-55, 58, 62, 65, 81, 90-91, 97, 107, 111-112, 116, 127, 137-139, 158, 190-191, 197, 199, 201, 208, 211, 218-220

St Albert the Great, 1, 82
St Augustine, 2, 34, 37, 67, 141, 160, 163, 183, 192, 200, 207
St Basil the Great, 21, 177
St Bernard of Clairvaux, 178
St Francis of Assisi, 5-6, 151, 171, 213, 218
St Irenaeus, 104, 159, 195
St John Chrysostom, 178
St John of Damascus, 178
St Justin, 158-159
St Thomas Aquinas, 6, 31, 38, 60, 67, 81-82, 109, 126-129, 141, 154, 160, 163-166, 180, 204
stability of creation, 87
standard of living, 235
sterilization, 71, 250, 253
Stern, Nicholas, 280-281
stewardship, 5-6, 32, 105-106, 112-113, 121, 133, 151, 170-173, 207, 218-219, 227, 270
Strauss, Leo, 40
subjectivity, 157
subsistence farming, 235, 242
suffering
  animal, 6, 126, 198-199, 203-205, 208, 217, 219
  human, 130, 188, 203, 205
surrender, 118, 209, 220-221
survival rates, 234-235, 260

Taylor, Paul W., 137-140
Teilhard de Chardin, Fr Pierre, 6, 58-59, 69-70, 72
teleology, 57, 114, 116-117, 127, 139, 185

teleomentalism, 115
teleonaturalism, 115
temperature, 3, 56, 272-274, 281, 283-286
The Canticle of the Sun, 214, 216
theonomy, 142
Tillich, Paul, 154
Tomasi, Archbishop Silvano M., 265
Tonti-Filippini, Claire, xiii
Tonti-Filippini, John, xiii
Tonti-Filippini, Justin, ix, xiii
Tonti-Filippini, Lucianne, xiii
Tonti-Filippini, Mary, 222
tradition, 1, 4, 6, 8, 29, 38, 40, 61, 66, 73, 133, 148, 154, 199, 209, 218
traducianism, 37, 42
transcendentals, 6, 147-149, 151, 167-169
Trinitarian anthropology, 143, 181-182
trisomy disorders, 25, 49
Truth, 162, 167

United Nations (UN), 223, 225, 232-233, 235, 239-244, 258, 260, 265
unity, 2, 43, 59, 61, 70, 73, 83, 92, 98, 100, 103, 105, 153, 176, 182, 268
universe, 1-2, 14, 16, 19-23, 29-30, 32-33, 35-36, 41-42, 56, 60-61, 64, 67, 74-79, 81-82, 84, 88-90, 102-104, 106-108, 110-114, 121, 127, 143, 172, 179, 186, 189, 195, 212
utilitarianism, 117

Veritatis Splendor, 119, 142
von Balthasar, Hans Urs, 147, 150-154, 166, 171
von Linné, Karl, 38

Walsh, Dr Mary, xiii
warming rates, 273
Wigner, Eugene, 22
Wilberforce, Samuel, 12
woman, 67, 102, 130-131, 182-183, 192, 225-227, 233-236, 239-240, 246, 259, 267

www.ingramcontent.com/pod-product-compliance
Lightning Source LLC
Chambersburg PA
CBHW021849230426
43671CB00006B/319